KT-468-190

CONTENTS

INTRODUCTION

Some years ago, when I was a father with two children and a mortgage, paying for a gym membership was out of the question. Whilst I was playing football at weekends and training one evening a week, I could only get moderately fit, and even this regime was reduced when the season ended.

To supplement my training I began working out in my garage using second-hand weights, a skipping rope I had owned since my teenage boxing days, and a punch bag kindly loaned to me by a friend. In time I was joined in the weight training sessions by my eldest son and so I added a basic set of weights and a training bench from Argos. By using these weights and running twice a week I maintained what I considered to be a satisfactory level of fitness. Later, once I started working at a gym, I continued running but had the luxury of using the gym's machines, weights and punch bags at no extra cost.

In the current financial climate it has saddened me to see how many gym members are no longer able to maintain their memberships due to loss of employment or, where they were self-employed, the ability to find adequate work. When members could no longer come to the gym I would advise them how they could maintain a decent level of fitness with very little outlay until they got back on their feet.

Cheap imports have meant fitness equipment does not have to be a luxury, and I am an advocate of recycling just about everything you need in order to get fit, as long your safety is not compromised: a weak and wobbly weights bench will prove unreliable if you start lifting heavier weights. Similarly, those old tennis shoes might be really comfy, but I wouldn't advise running 5 miles in them on a paved surface; after I did exactly this and was

THRIFTY FITNESS

IAN OLIVER

SNOWBOOKS

Proudly published by Snowbooks
Copyright © 2013 Ian Oliver
Ian Oliver asserts the moral right to be identified as the
author of this work. All rights reserved.
Snowbooks Ltd www.snowbooks.com.

British Library Cataloguing in Publication Data.
A catalogue record for this book is available from the
British Library.
ISBN13 9781909679986
First published January 2014

Other books by the same author:
Boxing Fitness 9780954575984
Fifty Plus Fitness 9781905005161
Punch Your Way To Fitness 9781905005314
Toughen Up 9781906727130

unable to walk comfortably for a week, I bought an inexpensive but reliable pair of running shoes.

Many people do not realise how easy it is to get fit on a budget; and, if they have always been able to afford to go to the gym, many of the questions posed by this book would most likely never have occurred to them.

When it comes to health and fitness I believe in never lowering your standards, and the fact you can't get to the gym doesn't mean you can't stay in very good physical condition. Likewise, a drop in salary does not have to mean a drop in your fitness level and whilst not all the advice I relay in this book focuses on exercises that incur no cost, the remainder should still work out inexpensive.

I have tried to convey information as simply as I can (hopefully as if I were speaking directly with you) and without using a lot of technical jargon. This simplified system has worked for me and the hundreds of people I have trained. I hope it works for you.

Remember…if you are currently unemployed or underpaid – you do not have to be unfit as well and there are also some additional benefits that can be gained from training at home as opposed to the gym.

These include:

No gym or membership fees

Your own standards of hygiene

No travel or parking hassle (or cost!)

You can train when you like and in complete privacy

You can have your own personal soundtrack

No waiting to use equipment.

The equipment I advocate using is basic and affordable so... if you are operating on a budget that precludes a gym membership or simply just enjoy training at home... let's get started!

Ian Oliver, at The Bob Breen Academy

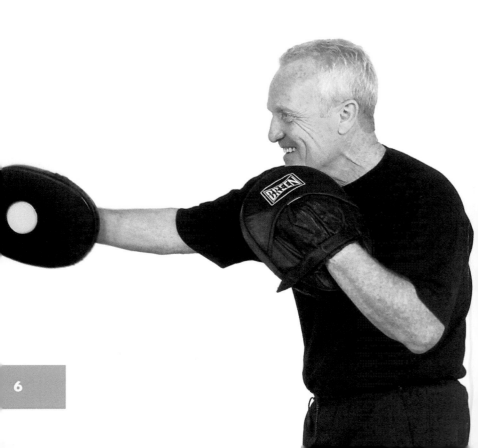

THE TESTS

SELF-TESTING

It is wise to establish at the outset of any training regime just how fit, or unfit, you really are. This is also a good way to monitor your progress without having to make complicated calculations. The following basic tests are possible with minimal equipment.

BLOOD PRESSURE

You do not need to take this too regularly. Your doctor's surgery will usually get a nurse to take it for you so you know what the starting figure will be. However, many people find a visit to a clinic can bring on what is referred to as "white coat hypertension". If you want to take your blood pressure on a weekly basis then you will find a blood pressure monitor can be found quite cheaply, and taking it at the same time of day in the comfort of your home should eliminate unnecessary tension and help to give a consistent reading.

Tesco offer free blood pressure testing and professional advice at their pharmacy departments.

PULSE

While the blood pressure monitor will also give a reading for your pulse, there may be a time when the monitor isn't to hand. You can easily take your pulse yourself. Place two fingers on the underside of your wrist or the side of your neck until you feel a beat. Count for 1 minute. Alternatively, count for 30 seconds and multiply by two.

Your pulse is a pretty accurate barometer of your fitness. The more you exercise, the lower your pulse should become at rest.

For the above reason, try to take your pulse just after you wake up, before eating or drinking anything. Make a note of it and take it at frequent intervals during your training routine, but always at the same time of day for a reliable, informative check.

WEIGHT

Not an important statistic, unless you are really trying to lose a lot of excess weight. Always use the same scales: they might not be scientifically accurate, but at least they will be consistent. Always weigh yourself at the same time of day, again for consistency. Everybody gets heavier by later in the day, so cheer yourself up with an early morning weigh-in. Try to only weigh yourself once a week. I consider it the least important statistic – the way your clothes fit is a much more useful indication of progress.

WAIST AND HIPS

All you will need for this is a tape measure. Take the waist reading at navel level and the hips at the widest part. Again, once a week is sufficient. Those with more weight around the waist than the hips are at a greater risk of lifestyle-related diseases such as heart disease and diabetes than those with more weight around the hips.

The calculation is simple maths. Divide your waist measurement by your hip measurement. Below are some example calculations:

34 waist & 38 hips = 0.89

44 waist & 40 hips = 1.1

Which means:

	Acceptable	**Unacceptable**
Male	< 0.94	> 0.95
Female	< 0.84	> 0.85

ONE MILE RUN

Any watch will be accurate enough for this. Time yourself and mark it down, then see if you can beat that time on your next outing. If you have to walk part of the way this will be reflected in your result and, hopefully, inspire you to get fit enough to at least finish the full mile.

PRESS-UPS

If you are too unfit to execute one full press-up (hands under shoulders, lowering the nose to an inch off the floor, slowly returning to the start position), and I have trained quite a few people who could not, then go for the "box" press-up until you can progress to the "full" press-up. Whichever type you do – beat your best on your next session.

Different journals and text-books give different standards for press-ups, but 50 full press-ups is generally considered excellent – so if you can't manage 5 full press-ups it may be time to start some structured strength training.

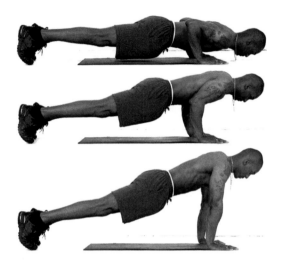

CURL-UPS

As with press-ups you are looking to perform more repetitions than last time. Nigel Benn, the former world middleweight champion boxer, was reputed to perform at least 500-1000 'sit-ups' a day, as his abdominal muscles attested. Be satisfied for 25 full repetitions to start with.

See 'Abdominals'.

WHAT KIND OF TRAINING?

RUNNING V WEIGHT TRAINING

It is a common mistake to assume that aerobic fitness, achieved by what are usually described as 'cardiovascular exercises' such as running and cycling, is the best way to achieve cardiovascular fitness, which is fitness of the heart, lungs and blood circulation.

The importance of resistance training in this aspect should not be underrated. Weight training can prove equally beneficial in enhancing your cardiovascular fitness. Running, cycling and other exercise generally regarded as 'cardiovascular' will enhance aerobic conditioning, but to improve and maintain cardiovascular health a combination of both is ideal.

EXERCISE
EQUIPMENT

CRUCIAL:

Weights, Bench or Box, Swiss Ball, Skipping Rope, Water Bottle

OPTIONAL:

Medicine Ball, Punchbag, Mat, Step Box, Timer, Press-up Stands

WEIGHTS

All you need for a basic home weight training kit is:

Heavier dumbbells for large muscle group (chest, back, legs) exercises.

Light dumbbells for small muscle group (such as arms) exercises.

If you are buying weights for your home there are some obvious factors to consider. I would personally advocate dumbbells for home use as opposed to barbells, which are bulkier when it comes to transporting them from one place to another.

How strong are you? You do not want to buy something you cannot easily lift from the floor, or that makes you struggle on the most basic exercises.

How strong is your floor? If you live in a flat and have downstairs neighbours they will not thank you if they are subjected to the sound of your efforts reverberating above their heads.

What kind of flooring will you be working on? Cast-iron weights can mark or damage a wooden/laminated floor, so will vinyl or rubber-covered dumbbells be a better option?

Storage consideration. A pair of dumbbells are certainly more easy to stash away than a five or six foot barbell, and a lot less likely to trip somebody up.

Cost. The whole object of this book is to show that you can get fit inexpensively. The required dumbbells, one pair light, one pair heavier, is attainable at reasonable cost by buying the type with interchangeable plates and 'spinlock' fasteners to retain the plates.

There are various sources of competitively priced equipment, but I have simply chosen Argos as I realise most people have a store within reach, at which they can pick their weights up, thereby keeping down the cost of home delivery.

Pro Power Vinyl Dumbbell Set £16.99 (total weight 15k).

Cast Iron Dumbbells Set 17k total price **£20.99** from Tesco Direct (collect from selected stores). Consists of 2 dumbbells each fitted with 2x 1k plates and 2x2.5k plates.. This allows by differing combinations 3 sets of dumbbells weighing 7k, 5k or 2k.

York cast-iron Dumbbell Set £19.99 (total weight 15k). Each dumbbell is fitted with 6 discs, allowing for more combinations than the Pro Power, but at **£7** dearer, will you need this?

Also worth considering:

York cast-iron Dumbbell Set £27.99 (total weight 20k). On the same date as above I found a second-hand set of this description for sale on Ebay at an asking price of **£6.50**. A similar set was priced at **£15** on Loot.com.

Ebay or Gumtree.com and other similar sites are worth examining for second-hand weights, as are the free newspapers you would normally recycle after a cursory glance. Items in your local press may be easier as they are like to be reasonably near you for pick-up. It is usually after the New Year period these things start to appear in these periodicals as that well-intentioned New Year resolution fades slowly away and the weights are now regarded as excess clutter. Boot sales are another likely source. Never forget that second-hand weights, unlike motor cars, are as good as new ones. My local paper advertises a York chrome 15k dumbbell set (**£39.99** new) for £20.

You can often find cheaper dumbbells online but, as with the eBay offer above, you will have to pay postage (hardly any company will post weights for under **£5** postage), or drive to collect, as it is unlikely you will carry them home on a bus or train, and highly unlikely on foot (unless you feel the desire to jump straight into some very serious training).

PRONE EXERCISES – BENCH OR BALL?

If the amount of weight you will be using, as I'd advise, is around 8k dumbbells, then a Swiss Ball will be fine. By using the ball, as opposed to using a weights bench, you will introduce an element of motor skill, balancing on the ball while lifting the weights. If you have never used weights before, or only used them a few times, working on the Swiss Ball may provide an unwelcome challenge. I would rather people were familiar with using the Swiss Ball before embarking on a weight training regime involving such an item.

WEIGHTS BENCHES

I bought the bench I bequeathed to my son for **£15** from a cluttered second-hand gym equipment warehouse (I have gone back to using the wooden box – see below). The cheapest new bench I have seen, as of this date, is around **£30** (the Pro Power Folding Dumbbell Bench is **£29.99**).

There are, however, many advertised on eBay – the drawback being you will, in all the cases stated below, have to pick them up yourself. If you decide to go down this route it should still (even with fuel costs) work out cheaper.

The following are examples from eBay:

Everlast bench £20

York bench & various weights £26

SWISS BALLS

I would advocate buying a Swiss Ball, even if you buy, or already own, a bench. The exercises shown using the Swiss Ball in the "Core Fitness" section make it an essential piece of relatively inexpensive equipment.

If you shop around you can pick these up at a very reasonable price. I haven't recommended the second-hand route with this article for two reasons:

They can be bought cheaply new (mine cost **£5** from Tesco, with pump, but I wish I'd paid a little more as the quality is quite poor).

A second-hand ball may have a defect, such as a thin incision on the surface which could cause it to burst; if you were lying on it holding a pair of dumbbells this would prove to be disastrous. Many of these balls claim to be "anti-burst", but I have witnessed an expensive ball burst — mercifully when nobody was using weights at the time.

Reebok £7.99 (from Argos)

Fitness First Gym Ball and Pump (from Tesco) **£12.99**

Amazon Gym ball £15 , pump **£5.49** (free delivery)

Tesco Gym Ball Basic **£4**, regular **£5** (includes pump)

Gymnic Fitball, pump and DVD for **£8** plus **£5** postage (Physiosupplies.com).

SIZING YOUR SWISS BALL

The following is a general guide used by most Swiss Ball retailers, and I have found it to be fairly reliable. Maximum weight is set at 300kg.

User's Height	Ball Size
4' 8" - 5' 5" /. 140 - 160 cm)	55cm
5' 6" - 6' 0" / 165 - 185 cm)	65cm
6' plus	75 cm

SKIPPING ROPES

Skipping ropes are just about the best value for money when it comes down to improving your fitness. See the chapter on "Skipping" for detail on rope size and type. Even if the "ropes" are composed of plastic, wire, plastic beads or polythene tubing, they are still referred to as ropes. I have tried to give a variety of different materials as it is often wise to try all types to see which variety of rope suits you best.

Osaka Speed Rope £3.99 (from Amazon, free delivery)

Golds Gym £6.50 (from Amazon)

York Speed Rope £5.50 (from Amazon)

Ampro Speed Rope £3 (from Sugarrays postal charge **£2.50**)

Reebok Speed Rope £7 (from Sugarrays)

Davina Deluxe £4.99 (from Argos)

Reebok Pro Speed £7.99 (from Argos)

PUNCH BAGS & GLOVES

While this is not a crucial ingredient as far as fitness goes, a punch bag can, nevertheless, help you get into terrific shape and can give you a dynamic workout. If you shop around they can be picked up fairly cheaply. As with weights, a second-hand punch bag is just as good as a new one. The bag does not have to be leather, which will work out expensive; you will get just as good a result with a vinyl or canvas covered bag. Don't forget you will need a hook or bracket to suspend it from. Check out your local newspaper and second-hand sales sites.

For buying gloves and wraps see full details in "The Punchbag Workout".

PUNCHBAGS

Preloved (second-hand site) BBE 4 foot punch bag plus wall bracket **£30**

Argos **3' bag and mitts £24.99**

Tesco **2' punch bag £26.99**

BBE punch bag bracket (from Tesco) **£16.99**

Various sites offer new **3' punchbags** for around **£30**, eBay has a total of 156 punch bags on offer, including several vinyl bags and one canvas bag at **£15** each.

GLOVES AND WRAPS

As I have stressed in "The Punchbag Workout", anything less than leather gloves is likely to be a false economy, vinyl gloves are unworthy of consideration. Protect your hands further by adding wraps, which are a good low-cost investment. Details on how to apply wraps is included in "The Punchbag Workout".

Lonsdale leather bag mitts £11.99

Pro Box Standard bag mitts £11- £13.00

BBE & Lonsdale hand wraps both £4.50

Pro Box crepe bandage £1.50

MEDICINE BALLS

An "old school" training stalwart that has made a deserved comeback, a really useful aid to any strength training programme. New medicine balls, whether rubber or leather are relatively expensive and it is probably worth looking around for a second-hand ball.

Tesco **BBE 4k medicine ball £19.99**

Argos **3k leather medicine ball £18.95**

Amazon.co.uk **3k rubber medicine ball £17.99**

Ebay lists over 700 varieties starting at around **£5**

EXERCISE MAT

If you are training in a carpeted room you can probably get away without an exercise mat. You merely need something comfortable to lie on while exercising and stretching. Even an off-cut of carpet will suffice.

STEP BOX

Useful not only for step-ups, box jumps and other lower body exercises but can also be used for various prone exercises for the upper body.

Step Box £14.99 (from Tesco Value Range)

RUBBER EXERCISE TUBING

These rubber tubes with a handle at either end are extremely versatile but relatively inexpensive. They take up very little space and by hooking them around solid home fixtures you can perform various pushing and pulling exercises. They are colour-coded according to how much resistance they will give: black tubing is usually the maximum resistance. Standing on one end of the tube (they are extremely durable) allows you to perform bicep curls; standing on the centre allows you to do squats. There are a great number of instruction books on their usage (get them from your local library). There is also a wealth of demonstration videos on YouTube.

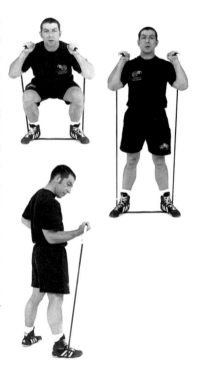

D.I.Y FITNESS EQUIPMENT – THE WOODEN BOX

With basic hunter/gatherer or carpentry skills it is not too difficult to locate or assemble a stable wooden box that can form a basic part of your resistance training regime by providing an adequate substitute for an expensive bench – a Reebok Deck or a step box. A strong wooden box can replace them all to a great extent, especially if you are sticking to a limited budget. My box was rescued from its final destination – the local dump – when the gym I was working at replaced these homemade step boxes with expensive Reebok versions. It is simply a rectangular pine box measuring 30" x 16" (71cm x 41cm). It has been joined at the corners with battens (you could use brackets) and a strip of carpet offcut glued to the top, which provides firm standing for step-ups and (minimal) comfort for lying exercises. I added small rubber feet at each corner of the box to provide a stable grip on indoor surfaces, and also on the concrete floor of my garage, which is its usual habitat. I have had it for about 10 years and I gave it a sanding and a coat of varnish this year as it was looking sadly in need of preservation. I have found placing an offcut of carpet underneath it makes it completely stable.

If you can afford the **Tesco Value Range Step Box** for **£14.99** you may consider that a more viable (and lightweight) option.

See "The Wooden Box Workout".

TIMER

If you are going to work to an allotted time on any of your exercises then you will require a timer of some description. Many exercises put you in a position whereby you do not have sight of a clock, such as skipping, so an audible device is more suitable. A cheap kitchen timer that 'dings' at zero, the stopwatch on a mobile phone or a sports watch may all suffice but I would always go for a kitchen timer as they are usually still audible above the sound of a pounding stereo or a pounded punch bag. I picked the one in the photo up at Aldi for **£1.99**, but for my circuit class at the gym I always used the very reliable (and audible) Salter kitchen timer (at the time of writing Amazon are selling a Salter 396 for **£4.44**). At zero it emits a continuous loud bleep, making it ideal for training in a noisy environment.

WATER BOTTLE

A water bottle is essential as training causes high sweat loss and it is vital to increase your fluid intake in order to prevent dehydration. Never wait until you feel thirsty. Sip water between exercises.

Buy the most basic supermarket 'sports bottle', i.e. one you don't have to keep unscrewing the cap to drink from, and just keep refilling it. Keep it cool but try not to drink ice-water when you train. Room temperature is the ideal.

PRESS-UP STANDS

Not essential equipment but nonetheless a superb, transportable and cheap addition to your home training apparatus. They allow more range of movement, while at the same time taking pressure away from

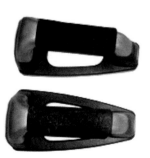

the wrists. Ideal for home training as they take up very little space, are extremely light and can be used on any surface.

The York press-up stands in the photo are currently on sale at Amazon (post free) for **£8.89**. Argos are selling Pro-Power stands for **£4.99**, and they are just as good in my opinion.

CARDIOVASCULAR EXERCISE

This is where you exercise and thereby improve the condition of your heart and lungs. The exercise I have selected require very little equipment or specialised clothing, as long as you have a reasonably good pair of running shoes. If you are already a seasoned runner then it may be worth skimming the early part of this section as I am going to assume everybody is a beginner.

The benefits of running:

- It burns fat
- It is guaranteed to get you fitter
- It will increase your resistance to fatigue in everyday tasks
- It can help you with most sports, such as football, rugby, tennis, martial arts and more, by virtue of improving your stamina and conditioning.
- It is free!

If you haven't tried running, whether on the pavement, park or treadmill it is worth starting out by jogging. Jogging is quite simply "running with the brakes on", basically plodding along at an easy pace, which is ideal for beginners.

JOGGING

If you wonder what pace you should travel at when you're jogging, it means you have enough breath to quite easily hold a conversation with a partner. Try to run at about 10-12 minutes a mile until this gets too easy, then pick up the pace. If you find your initial runs really hard, do not be afraid to stop and walk until you think you can start running again.

You may be used to vigorous running in such sports as football, rugby, tennis or similar, but you will discover that continuous, long running is very different, and you would be advised to start out by considering yourself a beginner. If you feel confident enough to consider yourself proficient when it comes to running – feel free to ignore the following advice aimed at "beginners".

RUNNING FOR BEGINNERS

Newcomers to running would do well to start out at a slow jog (at about 10-12 minutes a mile) and when this becomes easy, try stepping up the pace by small increments until you find the pace is "mildly challenging", which is a long, long way from "painful", which is to be avoided until you start to contemplate attaining a competitive level.

On your fledgling efforts you may find yourself fighting for breath and finding aches in places you hadn't experienced before. Do not be ashamed by having to slow to a walk to recover your breath or stretch your limbs. I am a strong believer in the "pre-run" short stretch, pictured below.

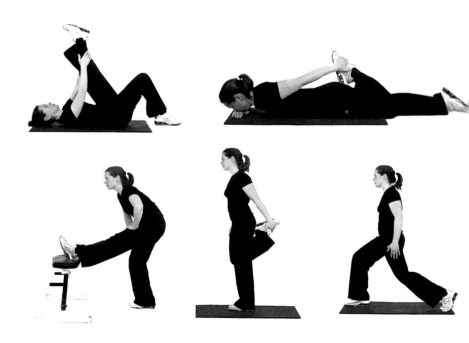

If you struggle at first – don't be despondent, most people struggle. It really does get easier as long as you persevere.

For your first "full" run, attempt 10-15 minutes, once you have warmed up. If you are setting out from home, or a user-friendly starting point such as a flat parkland path you think will suit you, simply run 5 - 8 minutes, turn around and come back to the start. Try to increase your mileage by 10 per cent every week. I would suggest 10 per cent of time as opposed to distance, as it is easier to calculate.

Once you feel confident enough to move on, pick a nice, flat course to begin with, ideally 2 - 3 miles, preferably in a traffic-free, and thus interrupted environment, such as a park or a towpath. Try to avoid granite pavements, which can be jarring, and if you are running in an urban area look out for paving consisting of tarmac, a runner-friendly surface. Once you have decided on your course start keeping a running log of how long it took, the weather conditions and how you felt.

TECHNIQUE

We should all have our own natural technique once we start running, just as our style of walking is our own. As children we needed somebody to teach us how to ride a two-wheeled bicycle, but nobody was required to teach us to run; it was spontaneous. There are, however, a few points worth mentioning.

* Keep your head up. A "head-down" style is likely to result in backache. It tends to be common in ex-service personnel who grew accustomed to running with a large pack on their back. Try to keep your head in line with your spine and your shoulders over your hips. Avoid leaning forward excessively, although a little is OK as running bolt upright is uncomfortable and unnatural for most people. Try to look ahead (about 20-40 yards), with the occasional glance down to avoid obstacles such as tree roots, or, when running on the pavement, something deposited by an ill-trained dog.

*Relax! Tension is something you are looking to avoid. A relaxed, loping style, devoid of tension, will make your running easier. With your arms bent at the elbow, let them swing forward effortlessly to and fro in sync with each step, with your hands and wrists completely loose. Do not clench your fists.

*Do what suits you. I have encountered people running marathons with flapping arms, high knee raises, head rolling and thought "how can they run like that?" But they are simply doing their own thing, and perfectly happy with it. Try to establish a style that that feels both natural, economical and comfortable, rather than attempting, in the early days, to stylise your technique or copy experienced runners. Be yourself.

ADVANCED RUNNERS

Seasoned runners should attempt to get out 2-3 times a week for 30+ minutes, with one long run of 60 minutes or more, rather than stay in the 30 minute comfort zone the beginners are looking to attain. It will also be beneficial if one of the runs includes an uphill element, and you can fit in a session of interval training (see below). Always try to beat your previous best time to ensure positive progress; if you simply keep maintaining the same pace, your fitness is likely to plateau. Try to challenge yourself on each run.

INTERVAL TRAINING

Competent runners' training can be supplemented – for running improvement, speed, fitness and as a diversion – by interval training.

This is composed of short bursts of sprinting combined with intervals of walking or slow jogging, termed 'active recovery' as the performer is preparing actively for the next action. This assists the purpose of recovery by clearing waste products from the muscles. At first the recovery can be completely passive, simply standing and regaining your breath for the next sprint – but not sitting or lying down.

Start out with short runs of 20-30 yards and try to gradually build up to greater distances, unless you are using this mode of training for a specific sport discipline, such as football; a midfield player should work on distances of 10-25 yards of speedwork (the training benefits of the long runs will provide stamina).

Boxers and martial artists in general combat or competition disciplines would be better off working on timed sprints such as 20-30 seconds work interspersed with 10-15 seconds rest, performed over 2-3 minute spells, to correspond with round/bout time.

SPEED

When it comes to the question of speed we are the beneficiaries, or prisoners, of our ancestors, who will have unwittingly predetermined if we will have fast-twitch muscles (good for speed) or slow-twitch muscles (good for endurance. Elite distance runners may possess 80 per cent of slow-twitch muscle fibre).

Everybody has both types of muscle but some, usually the quicker ones, have a greater proportion of fast-twitch muscle and the realisation of this at a young age usually shapes an individual's athletic prowess. Those with the predominance of slow-twitch muscle can, fortunately, still improve their speed by training the muscle fibres referred to as 'FOG' (easier to say than Fast Oxidative Glycogen): interval training can help with this, with regard to speed.

Many of the footballers I trained detested doing "doggies" (shuttle runs), and as a player I hated them just as much. It did not occur to me or them that repeatedly accelerating over the distance you needed to be quicker over – in order to improve your speed, and thus your game – might actually result in improving your game. To make significant gains will mean pushing yourself quite hard. To work effectively, interval training is usually a demanding form of training.

RUNNING SAFELY

iPods – wear your iPod if you think you need it to stave off boredom, but not in areas high in traffic (getting knocked flat by an articulated lorry will not get your running career off to a great start), or in areas with a dubious reputation where you may need to keep your wits about you.

Try to tell somebody where you are going, and if the terrain is tricky, and your mobile phone is light and small, take it with you; years ago when mobiles were the size and weight of a housebrick this would have been more akin to weight training, but now they are not much bigger than a matchbox it has become more feasible.

Look out for the twin scourge of the runner: the aggressive dog with the incompetent handler; and the adult pavement cyclist who has assumed by some unfathomable logic he now has the right of way.

DIET

Not too essential when you first start running, but, if you become serious, you may want to consider what foodstuffs are going to be beneficial. Training will require increased levels of energy that will only come from sensible eating.

Get a jump start with a decent breakfast. Even if your run is not until the evening, breakfast is paramount.

WHERE TO RUN

The majority of us have very little choice when it comes to selecting our terrain, unless you are fortunate enough to live near the beach or parkland with a woodland trail or sandy path it is going to have to the pavement, or tight to the verge on unpaved roads. It is still possible to find great, safe runs in an urban environment but that will probably mean driving or walking to the nearest park.

If you are running on the pavement try to find an area composed of tarmac, a runner-friendly surface, as opposed to granite which is less so.

A hypermarket car park on a summer evening or after dark if it is well-lit makes a practical, if unexciting, jogging track. Sometimes you have to settle for uninspiring surroundings when looking for a favourable surface; my usual run is to circle a well-lit industrial estate – humdrum but nonetheless practical.

RUNNING GEAR

SHOES

My advice would be to buy the best shoes you can afford from a running shop; manufacturers such as New Balance (which are made in Britain), Saucony and Brooks have, at the time of writing, reasonable models at modest prices, so it is worth shopping around. Cheap shoes from a run-of-the-mill sports shop will be, in many ways, more expensive, when you consider the wear and tear they could cause your feet, as well as the fact they are likely to wear out more quickly. Running shops are staffed by specialists who appreciate the fact that good service is likely to bring about repeat sales.

Look after your shoes, wash any mud off them before it "bakes on", and leave them to dry naturally, but do not feel tempted to put them in the washing machine as this will do far more harm than good. If they are beginning to get a little on the malodorous side, give them a large squirt of bacterial kitchen cleanser (such as Dettox), and leave them to dry.

CLOTHING

Comfortable cotton socks will suffice, and the same goes for t-shirts. Above all, never wear anything new; box-fresh garments can chafe in the most unlikely and embarrassing places. If you are even mildly suspicious a garment may rub or chafe in some places, then apply petroleum jelly (Vaseline) to those places before you start off. Nylon replica football shirts are another clothing item to avoid. They have, in my experience, caused the dreaded "nipple rash" more than any other garment. I have seen nylon shorts actually draw blood from the inside of a companion's leg, leaving him to shuffle painfully for the last half-mile. Wear cotton shorts only, unless you can afford a pair of those hi-tech Dri-fit, Clima-lite, Cool Max and a myriad other sophisticated garments that are two or three times the price of their cotton counterparts. They do a good job, but are not essential for somebody running 30 minutes, twice a week.

In cold weather, track bottoms and sweatshirts will suffice. A cheap waterproof will keep the rain off if you are an occasional runner. I picked up a lined **Puma waterproof running jacket** for the princely sum of **£6**, and a **Lonsdale knitted hat** for **£3** (on occasions **£1.99** in Aldi), for those really cold runs, from 'World of Sport', a great source of budget sports clothing. I hold no shares in this company, nor do I have any relations in their employ, but simply applaud their value-for-money sports range. Cheap wool or cotton gloves will complete your warm clothing outfit.

SAFETY NOTE

If the weather is foul i.e. snowy, with snow or ice on the pavement, foggy or signs of an impending storm – do not run! It might seem obvious but optimism regarding dubious weather conditions could prove perilous. Always err on the side of caution.

SKIPPING

A great low-cost cardiovascular training resource is skipping (or 'jumping rope' as it is referred to in the USA). Skipping ropes are cheap and the low-price variety are usually adequate to get a good workout.

If you can afford it my best bet would be the **Reebok Speed Rope** (currently priced at **£7.99**). I have used the earlier version of this one for years and, unlike some other plastic ropes, have never snapped it. It is available from Argos and the customer rating is 4.6 stars out of 5.

Really cheap ropes have a tendency to snap at the handle section of the rope and I feel a rope priced at under **£3** is likely to prove a false economy.

Other ropes worth considering are:

Pro Fitness Digital Speed Rope @ **£4.99**
Customer rating 3.4 out of 5.

Davina Deluxe Speed Rope @ **£4.99**
Customer rating 4.5 out of 5.

Nike Speed Rope @ **£9.99**
Customer rating 5 out of 5.

REASONS TO SKIP

Allows aerobic and anaerobic training. You simply decide what level of exertion you want to work out.

Tones muscle and reduces fat

Increases leg power and endurance

Improves co-ordination, agility and balance as upper and lower body adapt to the harmony required

Increases joint strength and, as in most rebounding exercises, improves bone density

Beneficial even when used in short intervals; especially efficient as a warm-up or cool-down exercise.

A refreshing fitness regime to condition the body for most sporting activities, especially boxing, martial arts and all racquet sports; in other words, those requiring the upper and lower body to synchronize

Provides perfect cross-training benefits for most exercise regimes and sports

There is no need to master intricate moves and manoeuvres to derive a useful workout; basic steps are just as efficient

There is something enjoyable in performing an exercise that is improved (in my opinion)) by using music to assist your sense of rhythm (upbeat music is an absolute must).

Don't be put off by assuming you are too clumsy, poorly co-ordinated or on the heavy side. Learning to skip is easy.

Before you make a start there are three major considerations:

- Length and material of your rope
- Surface
- Footwear

ROPES

(All skipping materials, whether rope, plastic, wire, leather and so on, are referred to as "rope".)

When you first start skipping, a light, inexpensive plastic rope is fine. What you must ensure is that your rope is properly 'sized', as pictured.

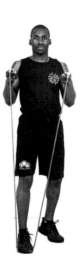

Ideally, a beginner should have a rope they can stand on with the leading foot, where the handles reach the armpits. Extremely tall people may need to get a "made to measure", bespoke version. Fortunately this involves very little expense; these can be obtained from most sports or martial arts stores. Shorter people can simply cut their rope to size with scissors or a craft knife and re-secure in the holder by applying a cable tie (available at any DIY store at minimal cost) or by simply knotting the end of the rope. If you are going to shorten your rope, err on the longer side at first; you can always cut a little more off – you can't put it back on!

SURFACE

Try to avoid concrete, granite, tarmac or similar extremely hard surfaces. The very least you are likely to suffer are blisters on the feet and sore calf muscles. The ideal surface is a sprung wooden or laminate floor. Skipping indoors on carpet, if this is your only option, is not quite as good as the former surfaces, but will not do any harm.

FOOTWEAR

Running, baseball, cross-training, tennis or squash shoes, boxing or wrestling boots are all ideal. Make sure your laces are securely fastened as a trailing lace will halt the rope's progress. If you feel the desire to skip in bare feet, try to ensure the surface will be user-friendly.

Other considerations:

Long hair? Tie it back.

Loose-fitting spectacles? Tie them around the back of the head to avoid watching them take a potentially expensive flight across the room.

Place your drink bottle near to hand. You may be glad you did this.

Skip in sight of a clock or timer, or set a timer with an alarm in hearing range (you will not be able to look at your wristwatch without stopping skipping).

GETTING STARTED

Be prepared to be a little patient with yourself at first. It will probably take a few false starts before the mastery occurs. If you mess up – take a deep breath and start over again.

START-UP POSITION

If possible, stand opposite a full-length mirror. It is important to keep your head up, in line with your spine, at all times. In order to maintain a good posture resist the urge to glance down at your feet to see how they are making out. Regulate your breathing by inhaling deeply through your nose

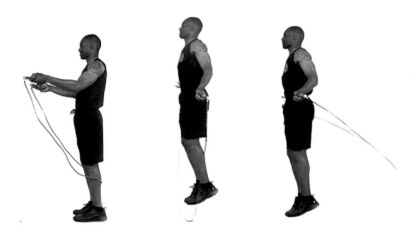

to 'get some air in the tank' – skipping can be tiring at first.

Start with the rope resting on your calf muscles, the feet shoulder-width apart. Start by bouncing lightly on the balls of your feet, with your arms completely relaxed. Once you have established a easy, effortless bounding rhythm, then, and only then, swing the rope up and over your head to clear your feet with each revolution.

You may hit your feet from time to time (every beginner does), which is frustrating just as you start to get the hang of it.

Training tip: once you are capable of making quite a few turns, and then the rope hits your feet – don't stop! Keep bouncing in the same rhythm, flip the rope back over your head, keep bouncing until you feel ready, then bring the rope back into action.

Once you have mastered this basic 'bouncing on the spot' technique, improvement will only come by regular practice. Do not despair if success is not instant. I have not had a single failure in the hundreds of people I have taught to skip, no matter how uncoordinated, lacking in confidence or unfit they were; some were more challenging pupils than others, but it is not exactly up there with learning the trapeze or ballet dancing, and they all learned eventually.

As you progress, start to bring your elbows nearer to your ribcage, so only the lower arms are revolving, and extend your thumb along the handle.

After a couple of minutes skipping it is worthwhile stopping and stretching your calf muscles **(see flexibility)** as they take a pounding during skipping.

ALTERNATE STEPPING

Start out in your two-footed bounding technique, then alternately place a foot in front, as if putting out a couple of lighted cigarette butts! Vary this by taking a double beat with each step.

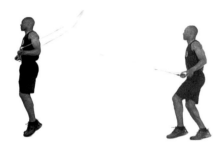

HOP AND KICK

Hop on one foot and kick with the other, each working alternately, the classic-looking 'boxer's skip'

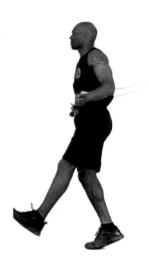

SPLIT STEPS

As you skip, starting with the feet together, open to shoulder width and back.

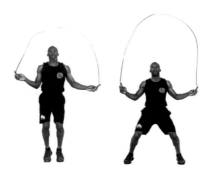

SKI HOPS

Keeping the feet together, hop from side to side, then switch to hopping backwards and forwards, really only a simple variation on bounding in place.

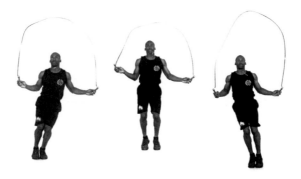

LEG RAISE

Work the abs as you skip! While bouncing on one foot raise the other leg until it is bent at a right angle, then the other leg.

BUMPS

There are other names for this but most people who skip know them as bumps. Finish off your workout

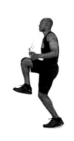

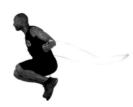

by jumping as the rope spins twice. See how many you can do in succession, make a note of it, then attempt to beat your personal best every time.

CROSS-OVERS

Usually easier with a slightly longer rope – the longer the handles the better. Start out by bounding, then cross your arms in front of you so the rope forms a loop which you pass under your feet with a downward sweep of the crossed arms. Once the rope has flipped under under your feet, bring your arms back to the start position. Takes a little patience to get used to, but looks impressive once mastered.

Training tip: when trying some of the more advanced moves it may be wise to wear jogging/track bottoms as opposed to shorts, as it is not unusual to "feel the lash" sometimes when you get it wrong (I speak from experience), so when first learning these moves you may want to "pad up" a little – jogging bottoms usually absorb any impact.

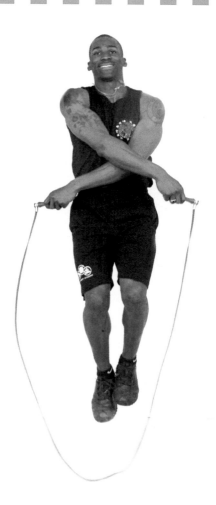

RESISTANCE TRAINING

If you are new to weight training, a simple explanation is that it works on 'repetitions' (reps) performed, whereby a certain number will be referred to as a 'set'.

Beginners would be advised to start with light weights and perform 10 reps to form a set. One or two sets are best at this stage. Once this becomes easy the participant should aim at what is referred to as a "10 rep max", wherein the first rep is easy and the tenth is challenging – *not* painful or discomforting.

Graduate to three sets and thereafter you may become specific, using more reps for endurance or more weight for strength.

Precede your workout with a 5 minute warm-up, a short skip or jog followed by a short stretch (optional – some swear by it, others find it unnecessary). Follow this by gently mobilizing the joints: ankles, knees, hips, shoulders and neck.

Always conclude with a 'warm-down' i.e. another 5 minutes of aerobic activity (skipping, jogging etc.) to assist recovery. Conclude with a 'long stretch' (see *Flexibility*). This last process should help eliminate delayed muscle soreness in the following days.

BASIC EXERCISES FOR WEIGHTS

Dbs = Dumbbells

1. Flyes – 2 x dbs on swiss ball or wooden box (chest)

2. Chest press 2 x dbs (as above) (chest)

3. Single arm rows – 1 x db, kneeling on wooden box (back)

4. Shoulder press – 2 x dbs seated on box or swiss ball (shoulders)

5. Squats – 2 x dbs   (legs and gluteals [backside])

6. Deadlift – 2 x dbs   (legs and back)

7. Bicep curls – 2 x dbs   (front of the upper arms)

8. Triceps extensions – behind head seated on ball (back of upper arm)

Possible additions:

9. upright rows (upper back)

10. front shoulder raise (front of shoulders)

11. lateral raise (middle of shoulders).

12. lunges (legs and gluteals)

13. seated bent-over raise (rear of shoulders)

14. cross-bench pullover (chest, triceps and serratus [ribcage])

FLYES

Lay on the bench, box or Swiss Ball, holding the dumbbells above your chest, maintaining a slight bend in the arm. Lower the arms out to the side level with the chest, pause for 2 seconds, then return to the start.
10-15 Reps

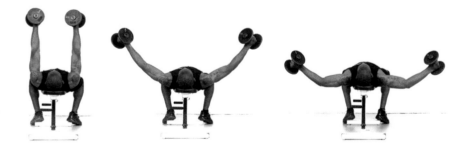

DUMBBELL CHEST PRESS

Lie on your back with the dumbbells held alongside your chest, then extend the arms fully. Hold for 2 seconds then lower them back to the start position. *10-15 reps*

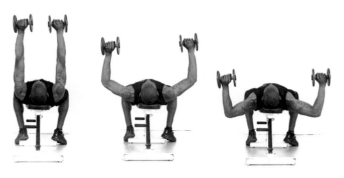

SINGLE ARM ROW

With one hand and one knee resting on the bench or box for support, hold a dumbbell at arm's length. Slowly raise the arm until the elbow is as high as possible, then lower to the start position. *10-15 reps each side*

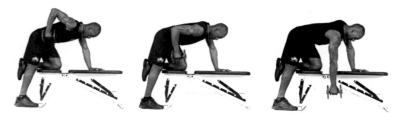

SHOULDER PRESS

While seated on the bench, box or Swiss ball, hold the dumbbells just above the shoulders, then slowly extend each arm alternately to the full extent of the arm, rotating the wrist just prior to the completion of the movement, so the hand faces inward. Pause for 2 seconds, then lower to the start position. If preferred, both arms can be raised together. *10-15 reps*

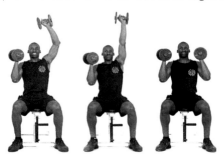

SQUATS

Stand with feet shoulder-width apart with a dumbbell in each hand, hanging by your side, in an overhand grip. Look ahead to ensure a straight back as you bend at the knees until the upper leg is parallel with the floor. Pause 1-2 seconds then return to the start position. *10-15 reps*

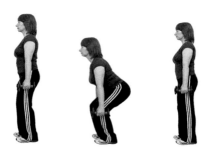

DEADLIFT

Stand with the dumbbells held in an overhand grip just in front of your thighs. Bend the knees as in the squat, then slowly return as you straighten the legs, keeping the arms straight, and drawing the shoulders back powerfully at the top of the lift, but maintaining a straight back. *10-15 reps*

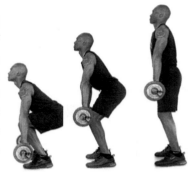

BICEP CURLS

According to the weight of the dumbbells and your personal fitness level you can lift the dumbbells alternately (ideal for beginners) or together. While seated on the bench, box or Swiss ball, allow the dumbbells to hang down by your side, then slowly raise them by bending the elbow towards the shoulder. Pause 2 seconds then return to the start position. *10-15 reps each arm*

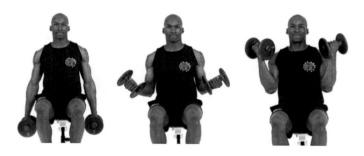

TRICEPS EXTENSIONS

Sit on the bench, box or Swiss ball with a dumbbell (a light dumbbell for beginners), at arm's length above your head, with your biceps adjacent to your ear. Reach across with the other arm to hold, and thus stabilize, the triceps during the exercise. Slowly lower the arm down behind you by bending it at the elbow, finishing behind your neck. Pause 2 seconds then return to the start position. *10 reps each arm*

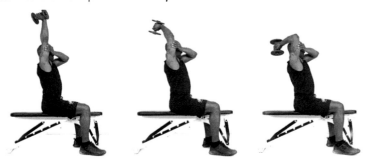

Note: The previous two exercises – "Bicep Curls" and "Triceps Extensions" – may be performed standing if it feels more comfortable.

If standing to perform these exercises, and the following three standing exercises, "Upright Rows", "Front Raise" and "Lateral Raise" – keep a slight bend at the knees to reduce any tension; note leg posture for "Front Raise" where Corey has his legs bent enough to assist a relaxed action.

UPRIGHT ROWS

Stand with feet shoulder-width apart holding the dumbbells fairly close together in front of your thighs in an overhand grip. Raise the weights until they are just below your chin (keep your head up to prevent facial/dental damage). Ensure the elbows are raised higher than the shoulders. Pause at the top of the movement for 2 seconds then return to the start position. *10-15 reps.*

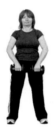 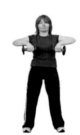 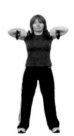

FRONT RAISE

Stand with feet shoulder-width apart with dumbbells resting on each thigh, held in an overhand grip. Slowly lift the dumbbells alternately to shoulder level. Do not raise the second dumbbell until the first one has returned to the start position. *10-15 reps each arm*

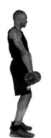 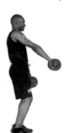 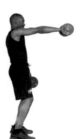

LATERAL RAISE

Stand with feet shoulder-width apart and the dumbbells held slightly forward of each leg. While maintaining a slight bend in each arm, lift them simultaneously up to shoulder height, pause for 2 seconds then return to start position. *10-15 reps*

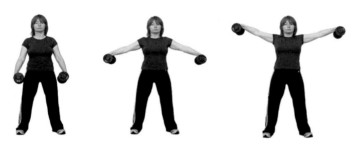

LUNGES

Stand with feet shoulder-width apart, holding a dumbbell in each hand. Take a large step forward in order for both legs to form right angles, while keeping the upper body erect and the head up. Continue on alternate legs. *10-15 reps each leg*

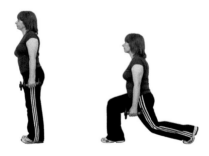

SEATED BENT-OVER LATERAL RAISE

Sit at the end of a bench or box, the upper body bent over in order to place the dumbbells alongside the ankles. Maintaining a slight bend in the arms slowly raise the dumbbells out to the side, hold for 2 seconds then return them to the start position. *10-15 reps*.

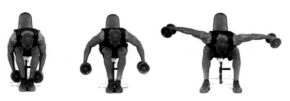

CROSS-BENCH PULLOVER

Lie across a bench or box with shoulders and upper back supported. Plant feet firmly to ensure stability before commencement. Hold a dumbbell at arm's length over the chest, with both hands flat against the end, supporting it with the palms and thumbs. Lower the weight in a gentle arc to reach over and beyond the head. Return the dumbbell in the same plane. *10-15 reps.*

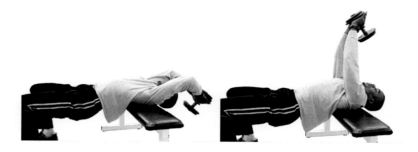

CORE TRAINING ON THE SWISS BALL

Core training – training the muscles of the torso which provide stability – has become commonplace in most gyms now, and although it was unheard of in this form, most people have been doing some kind of core training, such as press-ups and crunches, as part of their fitness routine for decades. The introduction of the Swiss Ball gave a new dimension to this kind of training. Although, admittedly, I sneered at it originally, I have come to use it in training with an increased frequency over the years. Most people I know who like to train at home own one. Mine cost **£5** from Tesco, and although it is adequate, I feel you do tend to get what you pay for with this particular piece of equipment.

■ ■ ■ ■ ■ ■ ■ ■ ■ ■ ■ ■ ■ ■ ■ ■ ■ ■

This item goes by various names, the Fitball, Stability Ball, Medi-ball, Physio Ball and the Gym-ball are just some other variations I have heard, but it was first introduced as the Swiss Ball, so I'm sticking with that.

It was first introduced by Swiss remedial therapists to assist primarily with back problems, and was treated with, at best, curiosity and, oft-times, with derision on its earliest ingress to gymnasiums. It has nevertheless grown in popularity due to the variety of exercises it allows and the benefits derived from these exercises. You use a numerous amount of muscles merely to stop yourself falling off the thing.

The extra effort required to manage the additional element of instability allows for core improvements both in strength and balance. The idea is that the unstable surface will place additional emphasis on the trunk muscles in order to provide improved spinal balance and stability. It takes a little getting used to at first and I would suggest using it on a soft surface to begin with – just in case.

KNOW YOUR LIMITS

Do not try any complicated exercises until you feel completely confident lying backward on the ball. In many gyms the Swiss Ball has been used as a substitute for the weights bench; this is all well and good, provided the weights are not heavy. If they are, it is far better – and safer – to use a bench or box (I've never seen anyone fall off a bench with weights in their hands, but I've heard cases of this happening on Swiss Balls when excessive weight was used). I have also known of a Swiss Ball being punctured: not a good scenario if your hands are full of very heavy dumbbells at the time.

I also strongly advise against standing on the Swiss Ball. Kneeling on the ball in a safe environment such as on a mat, or carpeted floor, is an aid to improving balance, but standing on the ball carries, in my view, no benefit that is worth the high degree of accident liability.

Make sure your ball is always fully inflated (the cheaper, thinner-skinned models, like mine, seem to go down more quickly) and keep it well away from sharp edges of equipment, tools or furniture.

GET THE SIZE RIGHT FIRST

The following is a general guide used by most Swiss Ball retailers, and I have found to be fairly reliable:

User's Height	Ball Size
4' 8" - 5' 5" / 140 - 160cm	55cm
5' 6" - 6' 0" / 165 - 185cm	65cm
6' plus	75cm

Most manufacturers state that the maximum load is 300kg, but although I would advise against putting this to a practical test, I do, however, know of a 30 stone giant of a man, a sports therapist, who uses his as an office chair.

■ ■ ■ ■ ■ ■ ■ ■ ■ ■ ■ ■ ■ ■ ■ ■ ■ ■

There are numerous books (see list at end of this section), videos and DVDs dedicated to Swiss Ball exercises, but in the following section I have provided a basic workout.

I have added a medicine ball in some of the exercises but it can be performed without a ball, or with a dumbbell.

THE EXERCISES

1) WALL SQUAT

Place the ball between a wall and your back and, looking ahead and keeping your body straight and bend into a squat position until your thighs are parallel with the floor, hold 1-2 seconds then return to start position.

Keep the pressure on the ball by constantly leaning back into it in order to retain it as it rolls up and down with you.

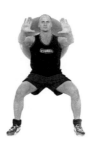 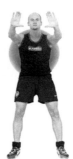

2) PRESS-UPS

There are two different press-up techniques which can be employed; both are, in my experience, challenging.

a) rest your hands firmly on the ball, ensure your body is straight (check in the mirror or ask somebody). Lower your chest down onto the ball, pause 1-2 seconds and return to start position. The slower you work the more control you should have.

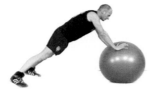 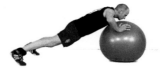

b) place your insteps on the ball and, ensuring your body is straight, lower yourself to the floor, pause 1-2 seconds and then return to the start position. To make it harder try to do this with the tips of your toes on the ball.

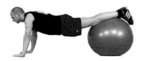 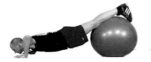

3) PLANK

Rest your hands on the Swiss ball in the same position as you would to perform a press-up. Contract your abdominal muscles but don't hold your breath as you maintain a stable position for as long as you can.

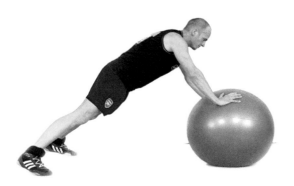

4) CURLS

Begin by sitting on the ball. Slowly walk your feet forward allowing your lower back to come to a rest on the ball. With just the tips of your fingers touching your head, progress to now curling your body upward, then slowly coming down again. Pause for 1-2 seconds at the top and bottom of the exercise. To make this a little more demanding, you can hold a medicine ball.

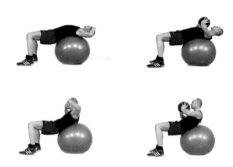

5) BACK EXTENSIONS

Lie on the ball resting on your mid-section. With your elbows out to the sides (as if giving a double salute) slowly lift your upper body, pause for 1-2 seconds, then lower to the start position.

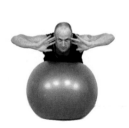
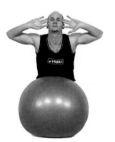

6) RUSSIAN TWISTS

Lay on your back on the ball in the same start position as curls (no.4). Fully extend your arms above you. If you do not have a medicine ball, football or dumbbell, simply place the palms of the hands together. Roll to alternate sides, coming to rest on the shoulder at the completion of the turn.

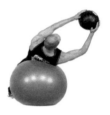 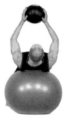 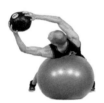

7) JACK KNIFE

These are also referred to as 'reverse roll-ins'. Start as if about to do a press-up with the legs on the ball (see 2b). Bend your knees to roll the ball toward you. Pause 1-2 seconds then roll the ball back by extending your legs.

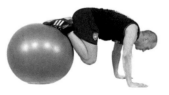 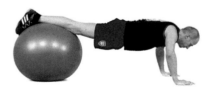

8) LATERAL CURLS

Lay sideways on the ball with the elbows out to the side giving a double salute. If this is difficult at first, try holding onto the ball with the lower arm, instead of bending the elbow. It may also help to start with your feet against the base of a wall. Once you are in position raise your upper body sideways as far as you can, pause 1-2 seconds, then return to the start position.

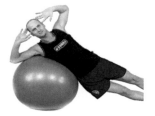 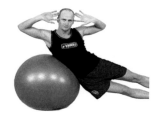

9) KNEELING ON THE BALL

A demanding balance test. Make sure you are next to a wall or a stable surface. Start with the ball on a judo mat or a large gym mat if this is possible – please do not attempt this where there is a concrete floor! Climb on to the ball with both hands and one leg, then hoist the other leg onto the ball, holding on to the wall for support if you feel unstable. Try to let go of your support as you come up into a kneeling position with your arms outstretched for balance, akin to a tightrope walker. Use a timer to see how long you can last, always striving to beat your previous best.

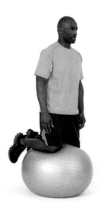

RECOMMENDED READING;

Lisa Westlake – "Strong to the Core" (Arum Press) & "Get on the Ball" (Apple Press)

Lorne Goldenberg and Peter Twist – "Strength Ball Training" (Human Kinetics)

Matt Lawrence – "Core Stability" (A & C. Black)

BUDGET BODYWEIGHT EXERCISES

In his book *Notes From a Small Island*, Bill Bryson related how his father would ask before any family outing, "Is it educational? Is it free?"

In this chapter I have asked myself, "Is it functional? Is it free?" I believe I can answer both in the affirmative. You do not need equipment to get fit, and I hope the following menu of exercises will confirm this.

There are 3 categories. You may want to exercise with these on alternate days in the interest of rest and recovery.

Press-ups plus

Abdominals

Back and Legs plus

The only pieces of equipment, all optional, are a box/bench and press-up stands.

PRESS-UPS

Ever wonder why press-ups (or push-ups, if you prefer), are easy when you simply stand and do them against a wall, but demanding to the point of discomfort when you start from a prone position? The answer lies in gravity; when you lower yourself down you are going in the same direction as gravity, so it is easy; conversely, when you lift yourself up, it is against the considerable resistance of gravity, and it becomes gruelling after a number of repetitions. The plain, if unhelpful, truth to achieving a good number of repetitions is straightforward: the more often you do them, the more you can do. Everybody knows they are demanding, especially P.E. teachers, martial arts instructors and drill sergeants, as many of us know well. It is generally considered that the individual will be lifting around 65% of their body weight, so somebody of 11 stone (69.9 kilos) will be lifting approximately just under 45.5 kilos, or just over 7 stone.

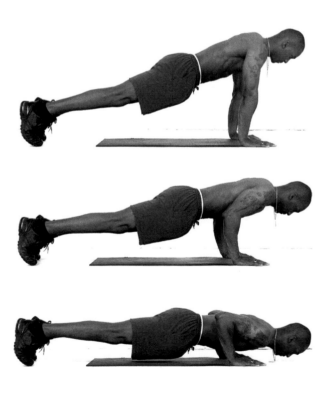

Press-ups are a good old-fashioned exercise for strengthening the upper body. They are, of course free – in that they require no equipment – however some minor equipment additions can, as I have attempted to illustrate, bring enormous variety and, in some cases, improvement.

The press-up is employed in most strength test cases as a decisive factor in determining the physical strength of the individual. The standard press-up works the chest (pectorals), the back of the arms (triceps) and the shoulders (anterior deltoids). Elevating the feet emphasises the upper chest; elevating the torso emphasises the lower chest. How many full press-ups you can do in one session is a fair indicator of your personal strength; it then follows the more press-up workouts you do, the stronger you should become.

Start by lying on the floor with the hands pressed flat to the floor, about shoulder-width apart. Slowly lift yourself up until your arms are fully extended. On each descent, try to brush the floor with the chest or chin, while at all times keeping the back straight.

Training tips: perform your press-ups side-on to a mirror to check for a straight back. Any spine deviation can thus quickly be corrected. Inhale on the 'down' section, exhale on the 'up' section.

VARIATIONS ON A PRESS-UP THEME

Each variation will make a slight difference in emphasis to help build a powerful upper torso. Those involving a Swiss Ball or medicine ball are aimed at providing an unstable surface, for either feet or hands, in order to use an advanced version of the press-up involving stabilising muscles.

FEET ELEVATED

Use a box, bench, Swiss Ball, kitchen chair, stout crate or lower stair to lift the feet.

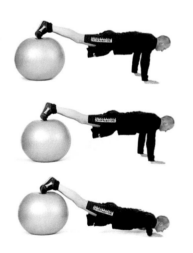

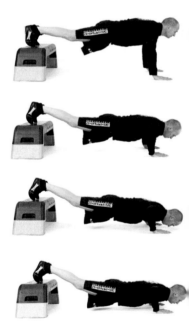

TORSO ELEVATED

Perform the exercise with a narrow grip using a Swiss Ball, medicine ball (substitute a football, basketball or similar if you do not have a medicine ball).

Once you have mastered this try one-arm press-ups with one arm on the ball.

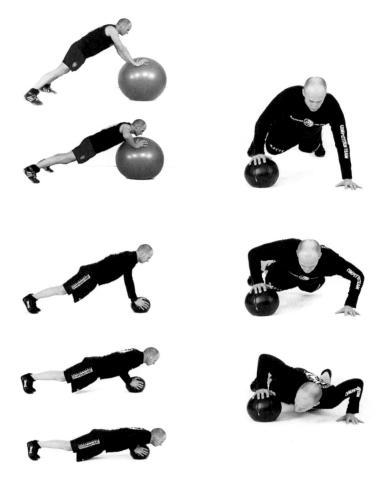

PRESS-UP STANDS (OPTIONAL)

Press-up stands are a cheap but effective way of enhancing your press-ups. They allow more range of movement, in that the chest can travel down past the hands, and at the same time take pressure away from the wrists. They can also be incorporated into 'feet elevated' press-ups. They are ideal for home training as they are light and take up very little space. While they are hardly a crucial addition to your home training (some traditionalists consider them totally unnecessary), in my opinion, at about a fiver a pair, they are worth having.

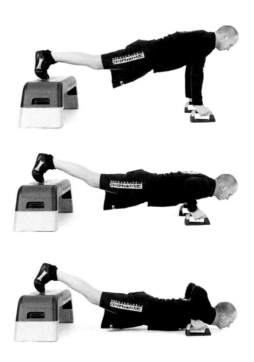

ROTATIONAL PRESS-UPS

After completing the 'down' phase of the press-up, turn to extend one arm to point toward the ceiling while the other fully extended arm supports the body as it turns sideways (see photo below). This will give the additional benefit of working the torso and shoulder muscles.

This exercise can be made harder with the introduction of dumbbells, but in the interests of safety, the dumbbells must be of the hexagonal variety. Do not try this with round-ended dumbbells.

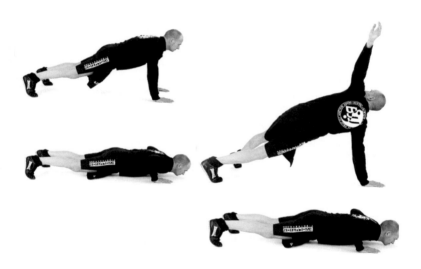

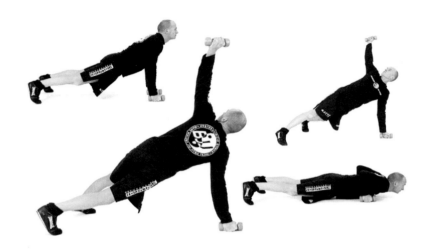

OTHER VARIATIONS

Performing press-ups with a narrow hand position, fingers splayed in such a way as to form a triangular shape with the index fingers and thumbs, will emphasise the triceps. A wider than shoulder-width hand placement will emphasise the chest muscles. For a challenge try "Clap Hands" press-ups; popping up high for a hand-clap before you make your descent. This takes a little getting used to.

ABDOMINAL EXERCISES

The following exercises are capable of being performed without any equipment, although a mat would be advisable. Exercises involving the Swiss Ball to work the abdominals can be found in the "Core Training" section.

CURLS (OR CURL-UPS)

Lie on a mat with your knees bent at right angles. Bend your elbows so your fingers rest lightly against the side of your head – do not clasp the back of your neck as this will almost certainly result in neck pain. Slowly raise your head until your shoulder blades (not your back) are off the floor. Pause for two seconds, and then lower to the start position. **Start with 15-20 curls, progress to 30-50**

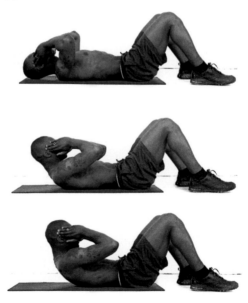

CRUNCHES

In the example shown a box is used to elevate the legs, but you can simply raise your legs into a right angle position, or use the bottom stair or a kitchen chair. Slowly raise the head towards the knees, ensuring your lower back stays on the floor. Start with *15-20 curls, progress to 30-50*

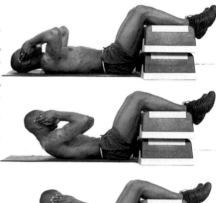

REVERSE CURLS

Lie on your back on a mat. Raise your legs, crossed at the ankles for stability, into a right angle. Slowly draw your knees towards your upper body until your backside is off the floor – not your lower back. Slowly return to the start position. Start with *10-15 reps, progress to 20-25*

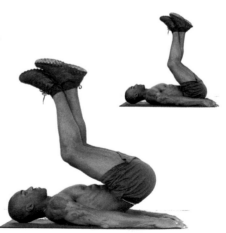

OBLIQUE TWISTS

Known aeons ago as 'twisting sit-ups'. Lay on a mat with knees bent and fingers resting lightly against the side of the head. Slowly raise the trunk, maintaining the lower back on the floor and twist the upper body so the elbow points at the opposite knee. This exercise can also be performed with the feet raised or elevated on a box or bench, which makes it slightly more difficult. Start with **10-15 reps, progress to 20-25**

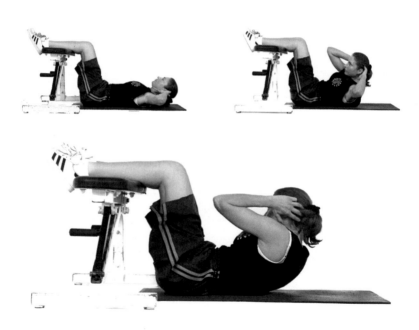

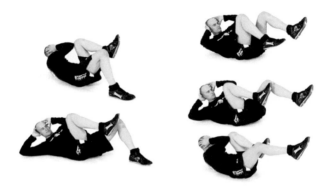

DOUBLE CRUNCH

Lay on a mat with your knees bent and fingers resting lightly against the side of the head. Slowly 'crunch' forward while raising the legs simultaneously to meet the elbows. Challenging but rewarding. Start with *10-15 reps, progress to 20-25*

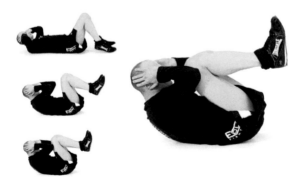

FRONT PLANK

(ALSO KNOWN AS "THE BRIDGE" AND "HOVERS")

Lie face down on a mat supported by your elbows and toes. Your arms should be bent at right angles, the elbows directly below the shoulders.

As with press-ups, check your form in a mirror or ask a friend to confirm you are parallel to the floor; try not to sag or stick your backside up in the air. Your head should be in line with your spine.

Contract your abdominal muscles but do not hold your breath; breathe normally. If this is too difficult to maintain, try placing the knees instead of the toes on the floor until you can graduate to the harder version.

This exercise targets the transverse abdominals. Have a watch or timer in view to time you. *Hold the position for 30-60 seconds, progress to holding for 2 minutes or longer.*

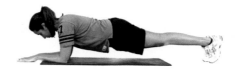

SIDE PLANK

The sideway version of the above, and possibly more challenging, rest on the elbow and side of the foot. *Hold the position for 30-60 seconds progress to 1.5 - 2 minutes*

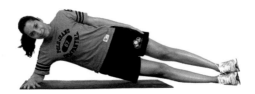

BACK EXTENSIONS

Lie face down on a comfortable surface; if it's not comfortable when you start, it is unlikely to improve after 10 or more repetitions. Place your hands close to your head, arms bent at the elbows. Slowly lift your trunk off the floor in a controlled movement, without extending your back, or holding your breath.

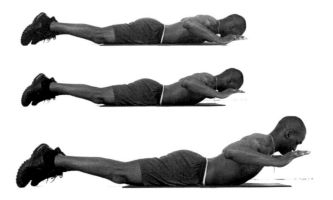

SQUATS

Performed as in the weight training section, but nonetheless still having merit as a weight-free exercise. If you have never performed squats with weights this is an excellent rehearsal for doing so, as it still provides leg strength and endurance. If the object of the exercise is endurance then a high number of repetitions are advisable.

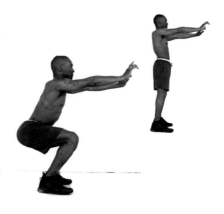

Stand with feet shoulder-width apart, slightly turned outwards, then looking straight ahead to ensure an upright upper body, bend at the knees until they are approximately parallel to the floor. The knees should finish directly above the knees. Beginners should start with the arms extended in front of the shoulders to assist balance.

LUNGES

As with squats, usually performed with weights, but as with squats a valuable weight-free exercise as it not only helps build leg strength and endurance, but has the additional benefit of improving balance and co-ordination.

Start with feet shoulder-width apart; keeping your upper body upright, step forward with one foot, bending the knee to form a right angle, with the lower part of the leg vertical, the knee above the ankle. The rear leg should also form a right angle, the lower section a few inches above the floor. Bring the leading leg back and repeat the action with the other leg. If you feel a little unsteady on your first attempts try spreading your arms out to the sides akin to a tightrope walker. Keep your head up at all times to maintain good alignment. Check your form in a mirror, if possible.

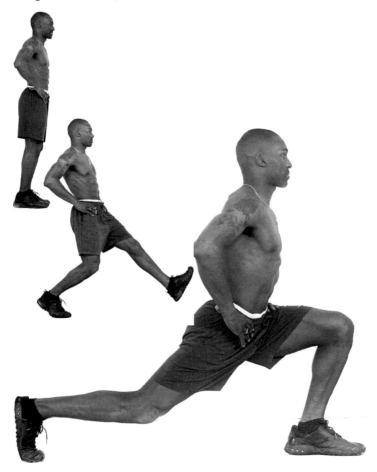

CALF RAISE

These can be performed on a flat surface, but are much more beneficial if using the bottom stair or similar. Simply go up on the toes, then allow the heels to descend slowly, going as far up on the toes as you can on each repetition. Using the stair will allow the heel to drop lower which gives a greater range of motion. Keep the body upright at all times. If these are to be performed on a flat surface place one hand against the wall for stability. Start with a low number of repetitions as the effect on this small muscle group can cause soreness if it is overworked.

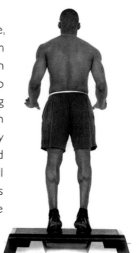

SQUAT THRUSTS & BURPEES

Both of these exercises have their origins in the mists of time, and are generally referred to as "old school" (I sadly remember doing them at school), but as with many old exercises, they are enjoying a new lease of life, probably due to the high amount of upper and lower muscles they engage. The latter is merely an advanced version of the former, making it slightly more complex – and harder!

SQUAT THRUST

Stand with feet shoulder-width apart, and then go into a deep squat with the hands on the floor in front of the feet. As the hands touch the floor, palms flat and fingers splayed to give firm contact, thrust the legs backward to adopt a press-up position. As with a correct press-up position, keep the back straight. Then drive the knees back to their former position.

BURPEE

The burpee, according to Wikipedia, is attributed to an American psychologist with the illustrious moniker of Royal H Burpee, who allegedly employed it as a test of agility and co-ordination. My old P.E. instructor used it for the same reason. Also, he despised small boys.

It is simply a squat thrust, with the additional demand that you stand up on returning to the start position; I feel 'demanding' is an appropriate term for this excellent exercise. The truly fit among you can insert a press-up prior to standing up.

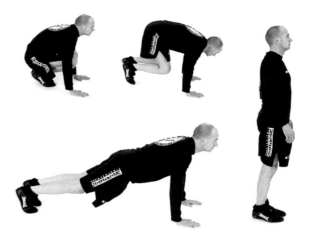

TRICEPS DIPS

You can employ a step box, but any elevated surface will do (the bottom stair or step will be perfect), and it can be used on a flat surface, only not to such a good effect as your range will be limited.

Place your hands behind you, with the heel of each hand firmly gripping the edge of the surface. Keep the knees bent (straight legs make it a challenge worth trying) and bend the arms into a right angle as you slowly lower your body, keeping the head up.

TUCK JUMPS

Start with feet shoulder-width apart. Go into a half-squat prior to making a vertical take off, bringing the knees up to the chest. Land softly with bent knees to absorb the shock. Beginners should take a few light bounces before "taking off" again. Start with a 30 second session. Progress to 1-2 minutes.

BOUNDING AND HOPPING

Bounding: place some low hurdles (small cardboard boxes, phone books will suffice) a few feet apart, then bound over them to land lightly on both feet, spin around and bound back to the start. Then try it sideways.

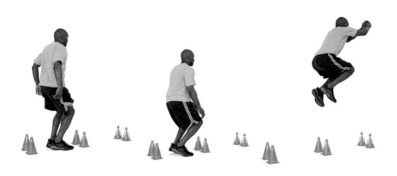

Hopping: as above, but on one leg, changing legs for the return phase. With each discipline start out with a one minute set, then progress by half a minute week by week.

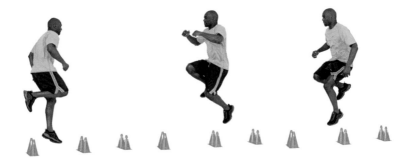

SHADOW BOXING

Although I cover shadow boxing in the boxing fitness section later in this book, I feel it is worth a mention in bodyweight exercises because it can be used in a relaxed manner to allow recovery after demanding anaerobic exercises, without the participant actually coming to a complete halt in the workout. While some may favour "running on the spot", shadow boxing has the advantage of employing both upper and lower body in co-ordinated movement.

For an optional version, which will, however, intensify your training, try the 'heavy hands' drill, which assists speed and power.

Use 2 x 1k dumbbells or 2 x smooth stones. To my surprise I have seen people using a couple of alabaster eggs which are both perfect in weight and hand-fit.

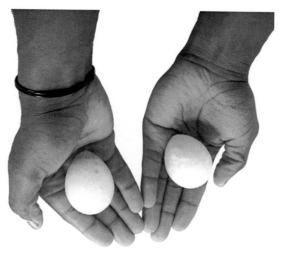

CIRCUIT TRAINING

Circuit training consists of training at a number of "stations" for a given time or number of repetitions.

The beauty of circuit training is in its flexibility and adaptability to the training needs, the likes and the dislikes of the individual. For example, if you hate doing press-ups then omit them from your circuit, and simply substitute an alternative chest exercise.

In a 'home gym' circuit you utilise whatever equipment and space you have for a self-built circuit.

As you are usually moving from station to station with a short break, or possibly no break at all, then it will be prudent to get the most out of your workout by allowing muscle groups a chance to recover. Try to alternate 'pushing' exercises (those which involve the triceps), and 'pulling' exercises, (which involve the biceps), thus avoiding tiredness, poor performance, or even failure, by these smaller muscle groups. It is also advisable, where possible, to follow an upper-body exercise such as a shoulder press with a lower-body exercise, such as squats. For overall fitness, a circuit can combine cardiovascular exercise with resistance training. Interspersing cardiovascular work between resistance stations allows the muscles more recovery time and, invariably, a better performance.

The main factors to consider when designing your circuit are:

- Time
- Space availability
- Equipment
- Your individual fitness level.

I find, even to this day, it is best practice with circuit training to work from a list, not unlike a shopping list. If you are getting the weekly shop without a list – would you remember everything, or end up the way my wife and I do, realising we have forgotten a few essentials? It is exactly the same with your circuit. Trying to remember every exercise in the order you want to do them takes a good memory – especially difficult when you are getting tired. Make a list, carry it in your pocket, or keep it nearby in order to move seamlessly from one exercise to the next.

Note: I would advocate starting with a low number of repetitions or, conversely, a low number of exercises. Starting out with many repetitions on every one of the exercises may prove a little challenging.

SAMPLE CIRCUIT

Insert the number of repetitions to suit your fitness level.

Exercise	Duration
1. Skipping or jogging in place	5 minutes = warm-up
2. Press-ups/ box press-ups	
3. Crunches or curl-ups	
4. Step-ups	
5. Back extensions	
6. Skipping or jogging in place	(as no. 1)
7. Shoulder press	
8. Squats	
9. Reverse curls	
10. Biceps curls	
11. Skipping or jogging in place	(as no.1)
12. Lateral raises	
13. Lunges	
14. Plank	
15. Crunches or Curl-ups	(as before)
16. Single arm rows	
17. Triceps dips	
18. Oblique Crunches	
19. Skipping or jogging in place	(5 minutes = cool-down)
20. Stretching (see Flexibility/ Stretching)	

The above circuit can be carried out at home using dumbbells or exercise tubing, a step-box or a box strong enough to take your weight, and a skipping rope. Add a timer (a kitchen timer or the stopwatch facility on your mobile phone), a small towel and a bottle of water to offset dehydration by sipping between stations.

As stated previously, make a list and this will help you keep a record of your training and give you the chance to chart your progress, a small, cheap exercise book would be perfect. After a month or two it would be advisable to make some changes to your circuit, especially if you are finding it now takes much less effort. It will be beneficial to try to make it a little more challenging.

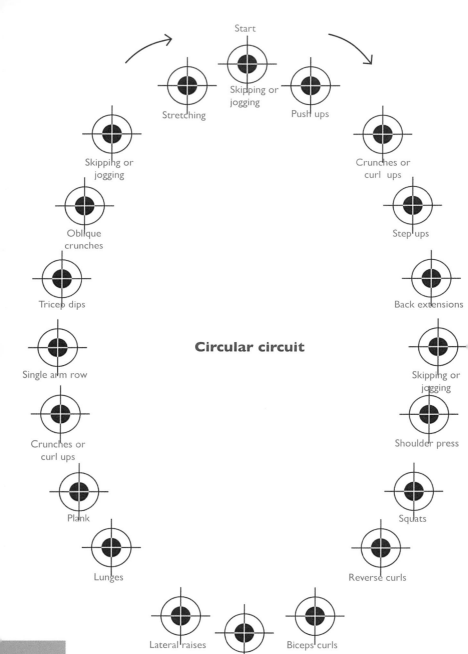

Circular circuit

Start
Skipping or jogging

Stretching

Push ups

Skipping or jogging

Crunches or curl ups

Oblique crunches

Step ups

Tricep dips

Back extensions

Single arm row

Skipping or jogging

Crunches or curl ups

Shoulder press

Plank

Squats

Lunges

Reverse curls

Lateral raises

Biceps curls

Skipping

OUTDOOR CIRCUIT TRAINING

In similar fashion to the section on bodyweight exercises I have asked myself three questions:

- Is it free?

- Is it effective?

- Is it safe?

An outdoor circuit should answer 'yes' to all the above. The only possible exceptions would be if the park with the equipment was in a highly dubious area or risky technique is used. As with all equipment, be it indoor or outdoor, there is always a risk of injury if unsound technique is used. Never use apparatus unless you know how it works, what parts of the body it affects, and how great a load or stress it is likely to apply. Most of the apparatus recently seen in parks, in what would appear to be an institutional drive against obesity, would appear to be aimed at people looking for gentle, uncomplicated exercises, as it should – since few of the users will have had instruction on use beforehand by a professional trainer.

Other outdoor items can be implemented to be included in your workout, often without obviously being fitness equipment. Provided the ground is dry, a park bench can be used for raised leg crunches, an inclined 'plank' and triceps dips, concrete steps can be used for step-ups and raised leg press-ups, a flight of steps can be used for fast stepping runs "Rocky" style. Performing body weight exercises, i.e. press-ups, squats, lunges, crunches etc will be far more beneficial in an open air environment, the sad news being – weather permitting.

Some parks (Hampstead Heath is one example) have a "Fitness Trail" with various items of (uncomplicated yet effective) equipment stretched along a woodland path. In other parks I have seen parallel bars, chinning bars, sit-up stations and hurdles. In an online search I found that some local parks have cycling and rowing machines, as well as other machines for riding, pushing or pulling – there is a surprising amount of equipment supplied.

Sadly, my first concern was vandalism (by the kind of sub-human troglodytes who smash up/burn down children's playgrounds), but close inspection of the park appliances gives the impression they were built by the same people who produced Sherman tanks – I certainly hope this is the case.

THE GREAT OUTDOOR GYM CHALLENGE

The National Trust is encouraging a more energetic use of its properties, as opposed to strolling leisurely through bucolic surroundings, in an effort to get more people involved in exercise. The program entitled "The Great Outdoor Gym Challenge" is based on research by The University of Essex which shows (according to an article in *The Daily Telegraph* 29th December 2010) that exercise in the outdoors burns up to 20 per cent more calories because the body uses up more energy keeping warm and coping with the elements, in addition to building additional muscle since the body has to deal with uneven surfaces.

The Great Outdoors Gym Challenge website (www.nationaltrust.org. uk/main/active) lists the following benefits:

(Their exclamation marks)

Training outdoors can burn up to 20% more calories!

Outdoor workouts are even more challenging – due to working harder with uneven surfaces and the natural elements.

Outdoor training provides the perfect total body workout!

Training with the uneven surface improves your balance and core skills.

Provide us with essential Vitamin D, which helps us maintain strong healthy bones, by retaining calcium, not forgetting a healthy glow!

I would endorse all these benefits and sentiments and add – it is free.

WOODEN BOX WORKOUT

Equipment Required: wooden box (or weights bench), dumbbells.

The number of repetitions is aimed at somebody with an average level of fitness. Adjust the number of repetitions and sets, and the weight of the dumbbells, to suit your own ability.

As with all workouts it is suggested that you start with a 5 minute warm-up, i.e. skipping or running, followed by a short stretch. The workout should be concluded with a 5 minute 'warm-down' followed by a full stretching session.

STEP-UPS

Start with 10 on one side then switch to the other foot, or simply step with alternate feet. To make it harder, hold hand weights or wear a backpack with a heavy weight in it such as a brick wrapped in a towel. *15-20 reps on each leg*

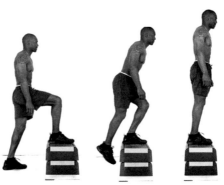

LATERAL STEP-UPS

As above but stepping up from the side as opposed to the front. *15-20 reps on each leg*

CALF RAISE

Stand on the bottom stair or a box with only the forefoot making contact i.e. have your heels overhanging the box while you support yourself by keeping one hand against a wall or rail. Firstly allow the heels to drop down then rise up on the toes, holding for 2 seconds before descending and starting again. *10-15 reps*

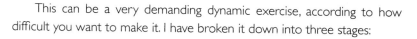

BOX JUMPS

To do this exercise your box must be not only sturdy but stable. Anything wobbly will simply not be up to the mark.

This can be a very demanding dynamic exercise, according to how difficult you want to make it. I have broken it down into three stages:

a) beginner b) intermediate c) advanced

Work to a set number of repetitions or a given time i.e. 1-3 minutes

a) beginner: stand side-on to the box, then jump sideways to land, two-footed, lightly on the box, then take off to land two-footed on the opposite side. Continue jumping from side to side, taking a double-bounce when landing on the box or alongside it.

b) intermediate: as beginner, but only taking a single bounce each time you land on the box or alongside it.

c) advanced: clear the box completely with a two-footed jump from side to side (see photo). To make it even harder use a second box or similar sized hurdle to complete two jumps in each direction, or hold small dumbbells.

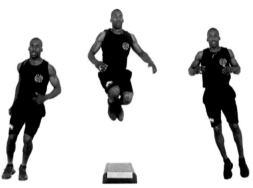

Training tip: Go easy on yourself and start with short time periods of working on this exercise, such as half a minute to start with. Build this up in 10 second increments until you can last for 3 minutes, which should be your ultimate target for 1 set. As you jump, perform a sweeping upward motion with your arms, bringing your hands up level with your shoulders. Try to land lightly on the balls of the feet at all times.

VAULTS

Stand alongside the box, leaning forward and grasping the box firmly on either side. With feet together, vault the bench from side to side. ***20-30 reps***

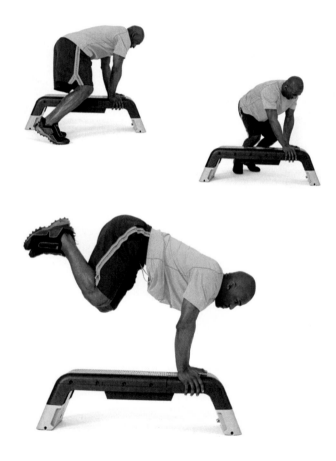

TRICEPS DIPS

Place your hands behind you, supporting your body by the heel of each hand, firmly gripping the edge of the box. Let your arm form a right angle as you make a slow descent, then straighten out fully as you return to the start. Begin with your legs bent at first but, to increase difficulty, try this with straight legs. *20-30 reps*

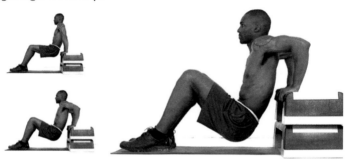

ELEVATED PRESS-UPS

As a standard press-up but with the feet placed on the box to place more emphasis on the chest. *15-30 reps*

RAISED LEG CRUNCHES

With your legs on the box, bent at a right angle slowly curl the lower body forward to bring your shoulders, not the lower back, off the floor. *15-30 reps*

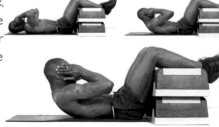

ONE ARM DUMBBELL ROWS

With one hand and one knee resting on the box for support, hold a dumbbell at arm's length. Slowly raise the arm until your elbow is as high as possible, then lower to the start position. Try not to give the impression you are sawing timber – go slowly. *10-15 reps*

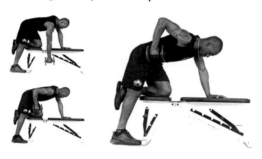

SEATED TRICEPS EXTNS

Sit with a dumbbell (a light dumbbell if you are new to this exercise) at arm's length above your head. Reach across with the other arm to hold, and thus stabilise, the tricep during the exercise. Slowly lower the arm down behind you by bending it at the elbow, finishing behind your neck. Pause 2 seconds then return to start. *10 reps each arm*

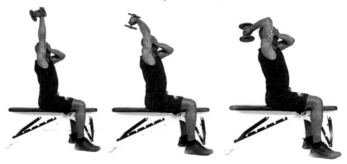

BICEP CURLS

According to the weight of the dumbbell and your personal fitness level you can lift the dumbbells alternately or together. Sit on the end of the box with the dumbbells hanging down by your side then slowly raise them by bending the elbow towards the shoulder. Pause 2 seconds then lower to the start position. *10-15 reps each arm*

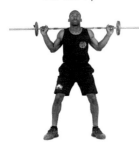 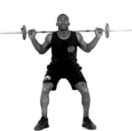 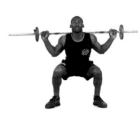

DUMBBELL FLYES

Lay on the box holding the dumbbells above your chest while maintaining a slight bend in the arm. Lower your arms out to the side level with the chest, pause for 2 seconds then return them to the start. *10-15 reps*

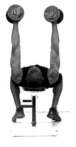 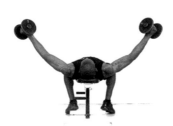 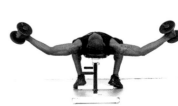

DUMBBELL CHEST PRESS

Lay on your back with the dumbbells held alongside your chest, then slowly extend the arms fully, hold for 2 seconds then lower them to the start. *10-15 reps*

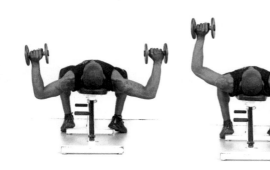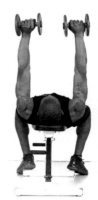

SEATED LEG TUCK

A great exercise for the lower section of the abdominals. Sit on the end of the box with your legs extended in front of you. Draw your legs back to your midriff. *15-30 reps.*

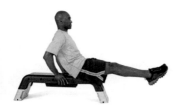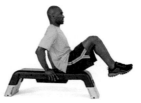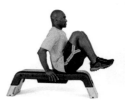

SEATED DUMBBELL SHOULDER PRESS

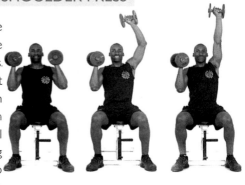

Concentrates on the medial deltoids, the centre of the shoulder muscles. Hold the dumbbells just above the shoulders then slowly extend each arm alternately to the full extent of the arm, rotating the wrist just prior to the completion of the movement so that the hand faces inward. Pause 2 seconds then lower to the start position. If preferred, both arms can be raised together. *10-15 reps each arm.*

SEATED BENT-OVER LATERAL RAISE

This exercise places slightly more emphasis on the rear of the shoulders. Sit on the end of the box, lean forward but maintain a straight back. Hold the dumbbells alongside the ankles, while maintaining a slight bend in the arms. Slowly raise the arms out to the side, pause for 2 seconds then return to start. *10-15 reps*

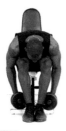
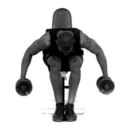
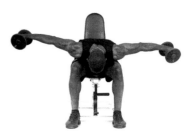

TRAINING WITH PUNCHBAGS

Apart from improving your fitness, any feelings of frustration or anger can be largely resolved by taking your wrath out on a punchbag. As you can see from the photo of the bag in my garage, you do not need a great deal of room to move around it effectively. A punch bag requires close-quarter work.

If you have tired of an exercise diet of cardio and weights then this kind of training can often prove a refreshing change.

If you have always fancied, literally, "having a bash", the following is a guide to executing punch bag work safely, and, with any luck, stylishly.

Your first consideration will, hopefully, be a pair of well-cushioned gloves, often referred to as 'bag mitts'. Try to obtain leather gloves: vinyl gloves tend to split and are invariably of inferior quality, and are, in my opinion, a false economy. A pair of leather gloves should last for many years. All they need is a wipe-over with bacterial spray on a cloth, and a squirt inside of them as well should kill off any unwanted odour. (This works with training shoes as well.)

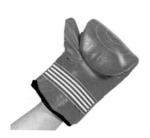 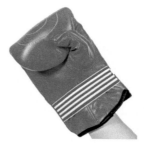

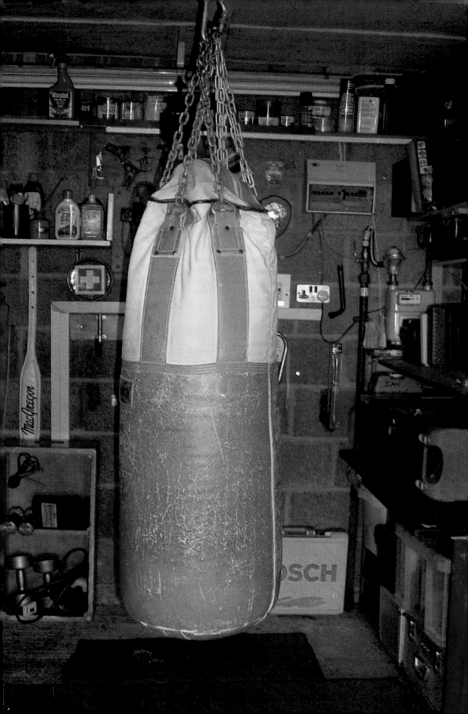

(See *"Budget Equipment"* - *"Punch bags & Gloves"*)

Once you are wearing them you will need to know how to form a 'fist' for safe hitting; although it may appear obvious, it is still worth emphasising that the thumb must be positioned as in the photograph above to avoid injury. Do not feel tempted to adopt the 'bare-knuckle' approach – the hand has 27 bones, many of them small and brittle. Always protect them.

Beginners, not surprisingly, feel tense when they start hitting something with force, but every effort should be made to encourage a relaxed approach since tension ruins technique and gives no added power or force.

There are only three punches needed to start with for a decent workout on the bag: the left jab, the straight right and the hook (left and right). Before throwing the punches, set yourself up in the correct stance. Imagine you are standing on a huge clock face with your lead foot, the left, on the twelve, and your right foot at twenty past. If you are left-handed, reverse all instructions.

At all times keep your shoulders over your hips. If you have to go forward, don't reach forward with the upper body: instead, move by stepping forward with the left foot and sliding with the rear foot. To reverse up, step back with the right foot and slide the left foot backward.

"Step and slide" is classic boxing footwork. It works well — and it looks good.

Training tip: when hitting the bag, at the point of contact make sure both your feet remain on the ground. Lifting either of your feet of the ground while actually punching lessens the impact of the punch.

The basic movements can be described as follows:

1. the front foot takes you forward
2. the back foot takes you backward
3. if you want to go to the right, push off with the left foot
4. if you want to go to the left, push off with the right foot

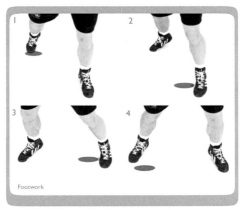

Footwork

SHADOW BOXING

Use the above footwork instructions, pausing to throw jabs, hooks and crosses in order to develop "shadow boxing", a really good aerobic workout in its own right. Always stop to throw your punches — hitting on the move is the domain of demigods i.e. Muhammad Ali in his prime.

Training tip: This advice is intended to assist in fitness training. Anybody who wants to learn self-defence or the art of boxing would be advised to train at an appropriate gym or institute.

PUNCHES

THE JAB

The left jab acts like a spear, thrust sharply at the target, hopefully delivered crisply and cleanly.

Push off powerfully from the rear foot. You must raise the heel but leave the ball of the foot on the floor.

Turn the left hip and shoulder in the direction of the punch-line which ensures the weight of the backside gets involved — arm-only punches are ineffectual and tiring.

Ensure contact is made with the knuckle part of the glove, where the hardest part of the hand — the middle knuckles — is located.

THE STRAIGHT RIGHT

Drive off the ball of the rear foot, turning the right hip and shoulder in the direction of the punch-line as you drive the right fist at the bag, hitting with the knuckle part of the glove.

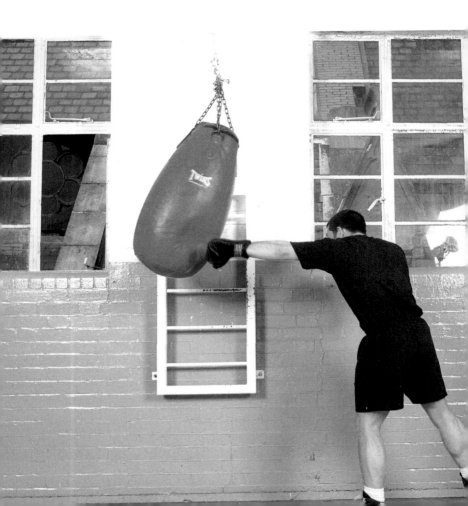

THE HOOK

Shift your weight to the side you intend to hit from, slightly turning the hip and shoulder away. Slide the back foot a little further behind the front foot. The narrower base will allow a more dynamic turn to create power, as well as making the manoeuvre simpler.

The arm should be bent at the elbow at about 90 degrees. The right hand stays close to the head.

Raise the left heel vigorously and pivot the left hip and shoulder powerfully as you slam the left hand at the target with the upper knuckles leading and the thumb tucked in tightly. After contact, withdraw the hand to the starting position.

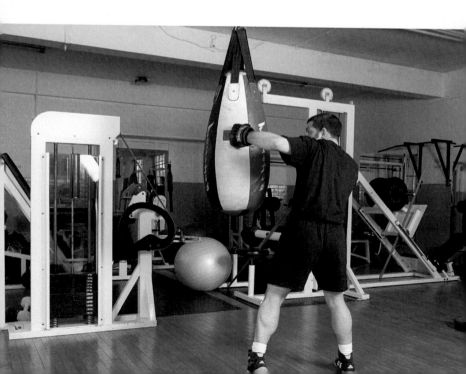

PROTECTION

It is wise to wear "wraps" for additional protection. You can follow the illustration here for wrapping your hands, or you may want to simplify this. As long as they serve to protect the hand this will be fine – there is no right or wrong way.

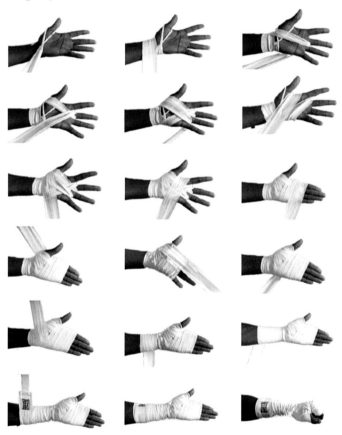

Wraps usually cost around £5, but crepe bandage will suffice if wraps are not available. Whichever you choose, wraps or bandage, remember to wash them regularly. Once your encased hands have been hitting the bag a few times your wraps are likely to become less than fragrant.

THE PUNCH-SPECIFIC STRETCH

Before embarking on a strenuous punching session it is advisable to stretch the most vulnerable areas of the hand, wrist and forearm. See below:

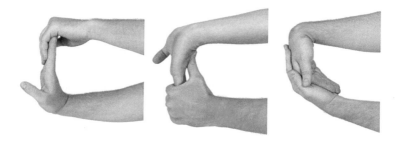

Ideally the best way to get the most from the punch bag is to work in 2 minute bursts, with a 30 second rest in between. If this is too easy, or you want to add more variety, try skipping 2 minutes (an ideal warm-up), then punching for 2 minutes. Try to get up to 5 sessions of each i.e. a 20 minute workout.

Always finish with the punch-specific stretch in addition to circling the wrists and shaking the fingers as if flicking water off them.

THE BOXING WORKOUT

The times and repetitions on the guide that follows are suggested as guidelines. Beginners should make appropriate reductions of time and repetitions. Advanced trainers or the very fit should make appropriate increases. Performing the squats and lunges with dumbbells, and the abs exercises on a Swiss Ball, will enhance the usefulness of the workout. Keep a clock or timing device handy for your skipping and shadow boxing.

Sip water constantly, re-stretch if feeling 'tight', and take a 1 minute break at intervals if you are unused to this type of training.

Training tip: you may consider accompanying your workout with some upbeat inspirational music, which is particularly helpful to achieve a rhythm when skipping.

Equipment required: punchbag, skipping rope, bag mitts/boxing gloves, floor mat.

	Exercise	Duration
1	Skip	2 minutes
2	Short stretch (chest, back and legs) & joint mobilisation	1-2 minutes
3	Shadow box (relaxed – this is just a warm up and rehearsal drill)	2 minutes
4	Punchbag – hit light and fast	2 minutes
5	Skip	2 minutes
6	Abs crunches	15-30 reps
7	Press-ups	15-30 reps
8	Skip – top speed	1 minute
9	Lunges with alternate legs	20-30 reps.
10	Shadow box	2 minutes
11	Squats	20 reps
12	Skip	2 minutes
13	Punchbag – hard, solid hitting for	2 minutes
14	Crunches	15-30 reps
15	Press-ups	15-30 reps
16	Skip	2 minutes
17	Fast explosive hitting on the punch bag	2 mins.
18	Shadow box	2 mins
19	Lunges (alternate legs)	20-30 reps
20	Skip (slow pace)	3 minutes
21	Long stretch including the punch-specific stretch, followed by shaking out the limbs, wrist circling, arm circling, neck rolls slowly from left to right.	20-30 seconds (each stretch)

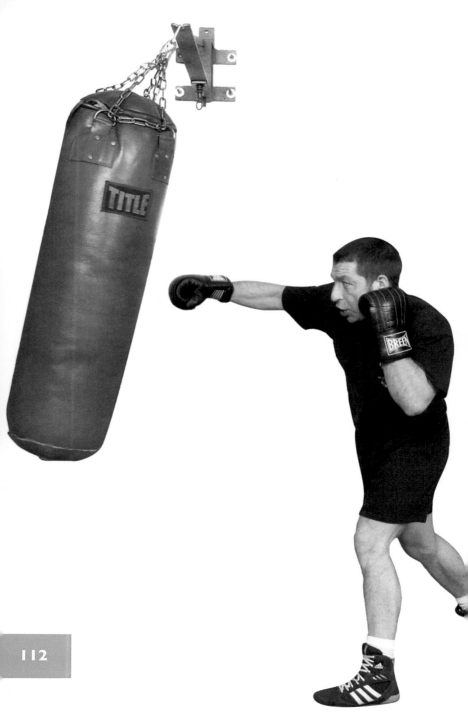

My garage punch bag is 3' in length and older than my grown-up children, but it does the job and there is just enough room left by my bench, toolboxes and assorted garage paraphernalia to work around it. I can, of course, dump much of it outside before I start if I feel I am going to need more room to work in. It hangs from a hook inserted into a wooden rafter; if you intend to hang a bag from your ceiling, ensure the structure and the hook are strong enough to take it.

If you cannot afford a punch bag just yet, try to get hold of an army-type kitbag, a large laundry bag, or a hessian sack, and stuff it with rags torn into strips (not in bundles). If it is not excessively heavy you will probably get away with hanging it with rope. Poundsaver, Poundstretcher and similar stores sell nylon rope for the somewhat obvious price of £1. If you don't want the bag to swing too much, fill the base with an inch or two of sand. If, once your bag is filled, it still seems a bit hard, try mixing the rags with ripped-up lumps of foam rubber. Do not be tempted to use sawdust. Even Mike Tyson in his pomp would have a hard time working with a bag full of this.

SHADOW BOXING WITH "HEAVY HANDS"

To step up the intensity of your shadow boxing there are some items you can hold in each hand:

   2 x smooth stones/ alabaster eggs

   2 x .5k – 1k weights. Anything heavier will slow you down too much, defeating the object of this element, which is speedy movement.

KEEP AN EXERCISE RECORD/LOG

One way to continually prod yourself into activity is to keep a training diary. All you need is a small, cheap exercise book, and a pocket diary – or a desk diary if you intend to write down all your weight training exercises, reps and sets. Every time you work out, write down:

Date & time (and weather conditions if training outdoors).

What exercise

How you felt (including any twinges)

Record of progress

If you are trying to lose some weight then also keep a food diary alongside your exercise diary (see "Eating Right"). You can roughly work out how many calories you have consumed by working out your intake from food and your energy expenditure.

Consider the amount of calories expended on the following activities: they will vary with your size and how much effort you apply. As an extra incentive in achieving weight loss, place an unflattering photograph of yourself somewhere that you can't miss it – on the fridge, next to the bed, taped to the cake or biscuit tin.

	Activity	Calories per minute (rough)
1	Driving car	2.8
2	Driving motor bike	3.4
3	Painting	3.5
4	Vacuuming	3.5
5	Sweeping floors	3.9
6	Ironing	4.2
7	Gardening (weeding)	5.6
8	Gardening (digging)	8.6
9	Cycling (easy)	5.0
10	Cycling (hard)	15
11	Dancing (leisurely)	5
12	Dancing (vigorously)	7.5
13	Golf	5
14	Walking (3.5 m.p.h.)	6
15	Power walking	8-10
16	Jogging (5 m.p.h.)	10-12
17	Running (7.5 m.p.h.)	15
18	Aerobics Class	8-10
19	Step aerobics	9-12
20	Running (10 m.p.h.)	20
21	Playing football (according to position)	12-17
22	Swimming (breast stroke/ back stroke)	6-12
23	Swimming (butterfly)	14
24	Swimming (crawl)	9-12

	Activity	Calories per minute (rough)
25	Squash	11-12
26	Skipping rope (leisurely)	10
27	Skipping rope (fast)	15
28	Rowing (leisurely)	5
29	Rowing (strenuously)	15
30	Badminton (recreational)	5
31	Badminton (competitive)	10
32	Table tennis (recreational)	5
33	Table tennis (competitive)	7.5
34	Lawn tennis (recreational)	7
35	Lawn tennis (competitive)	11
36	Weight training (general)	8-10

FLEXIBILITY

Flexibility is an integral part of overall fitness. Without flexibility our range of movement and ability to get the most out of our workout is hindered. There are two main ways we keep our flexibility and that is by keeping our joints mobile and our muscles stretched. If you live in a warm climate, or are in a warm environment, stretching will be easier. A cold environment is a restriction to muscular activity, hence it is wise, after a short spell of aerobic exercise, to mobilise the joints and perform a short, gentle stretch prior to vigorous exercise.

MOBILITY

It is advisable to gently loosen (mobilise) the main joints before a workout. This releases synovial fluid into the joint cavity which soaks into the cartilage to act as a shock absorber.

WARM-UP STRETCHES

Once the body is warm, it is advised that you carry out some main muscle group short stretches. This is not an absolute must – it will depend on your own personal preference. Research has found that warm-up style stretches can hinder an athlete's performance. However, most of us are not athletes and so a short main muscle group stretch can help prevent you from pulling a muscle. There has been no conclusive research (at the time of this going to print) that a warm-up stretch is not beneficial to the average person taking part in activity. Until such a time that research does prove this to be the case then the warm-up stretch is a safety measure that will give longevity to your training routine.

Warm-up stretches can be carried out statically (holding the position for 6-8 secs) or dynamically — this is where you do large movements, taking joints through a controlled full range of movement.

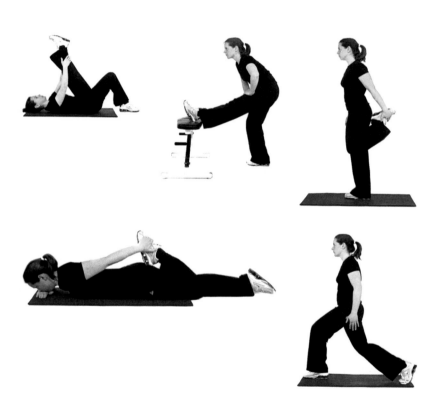

COOL DOWN STRETCHES

It is advisable to gradually lower the body temperature after exercise and at the same time reduce the risk of delayed onset muscle soreness (the dreaded 'DOMS'), which can set in 24-48 hours after exercise. Cooling down is also regarded as being helpful in reducing waste products from the system.

These longer-held stretches are important to everyone who is serious about improving their fitness. Post-workout stretches, as they are often called, come in various forms, namely maintenance and developmental stretches.

Stretches that maintain current levels of flexibility are the bare minimum requirement for a post workout stretch. These are stretches that are held for a short period of time I.e. 10-30 seconds each, and all they do is maintain the current level of flexibility. If your flexibility is not good you might want to do something extra in your post workout stretch.

Developmental stretching is designed to improve your levels of flexibility. These stretches need to be performed in comfortable and supported positions, so seated or lying is often the best option. Developmental stretches need to be held for slightly longer, so it is important that you feel warm and comfortable before you start. The key to successful developmental stretching is that you allow enough time for the muscle to relax before you increase the stretch. Hold a stretch at the point of mild tension (in the muscle being stretched). You are aiming for that tension to subside (for the stretch reflex to ease off). Once the tension has subsided you then increase the stretch to the next point of mild tension and repeat.

Developmental stretching can take anything from 30secs upwards per muscle being stretched. This needs to be carried out statically (holding still).

HOW DO I DECIDE WHICH MUSCLES NEED DEVELOPMENTAL STRETCHING?

Those muscle groups that are tight need developmental stretching. Often these are the backs of the legs (due to sitting all day). You decide: if you are unable to get good range of movement then the chances are that muscle needs some developmental stretching. A fitness professional can help identify which muscle groups need developmental stretching and offer you a range of positions. See below for a guide on post workout stretching.

THE STRETCHES

You can avail yourself of any number of books on flexibility which vary in how much technical information and detailed instruction they provide. I have worked on the basis that for now what you need to know is which muscles to stretch and how to stretch them.

I prefer a system whereby I start at the shoulders and work down, making a return trip to finish off with the neck stretch, which I consider the most important as so many retain stress and tightness here. For this reason I have added extra neck stretches.

You should have warmed up for at least 5 minutes prior to stretching — never stretch cold muscles.

SHOULDER STRETCH

Extend one arm across the chest, then pull it towards you with the other arm.

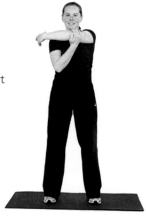

BACK STRETCH (STANDING)

Used in warm-up stretch. With feet shoulder width apart and slightly bent knees, hold the arms out in front, as if clutching a large beach-ball, while contracting abdominal muscles.

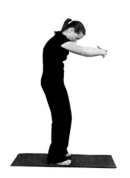

BACK STRETCH (PRONE)

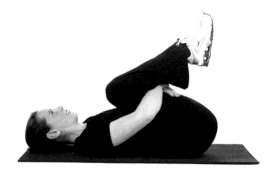

Lying on a mat, pull your bent legs toward you.

BACK STRETCH

(angry cat – spinal muscles)

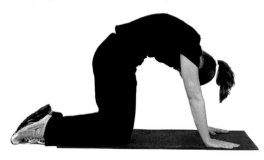

While on all fours, haul in the abdominal muscles while rounding the back like a hump-back bridge.

CHEST

Hold hands behind your back, raise the arms as you push out the chest.

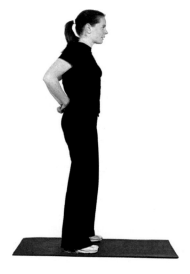

OBLIQUES

Stand with feet shoulder-width apart, raise one arm then list over to the side.

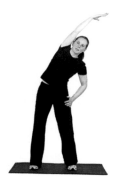

GLUTES

(the muscles of the backside)

Raise one leg, then place the other leg across it and pull the lower one toward you.

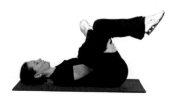

ADDUCTORS

(muscles on the inside of the legs)

While seated place the soles of the feet to touch each other.

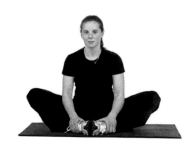

HAMSTRINGS (BACK OF UPPER LEG)

Standing version suited to warm up: raise your leg on a bench or similar surface and keeping upper body straight, lean forward.

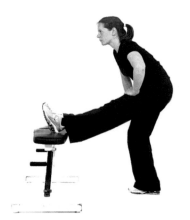

HAMSTRINGS

Lying version, suited to warm-down: lay on your back, raise your leg in the air and, holding your calf, pull it towards you.

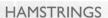

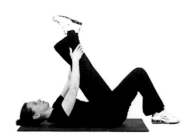

QUADS (THIGHS)

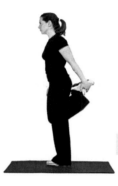

Standing version suited to warm-up: pull lower leg up behind you to touch heel to backside.

QUADS

Lying version: lie on front or side, then pull leg back until heel reaches backside.

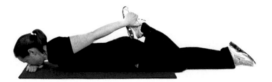

HIP FLEXORS (PELVIC AREA)

Keep upper body upright as you take a step forward, then lower the hips.

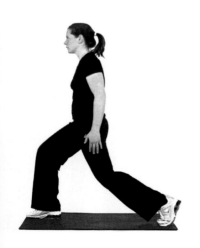

CALF MUSCLES

(gastrocnemius, the large calf muscle)

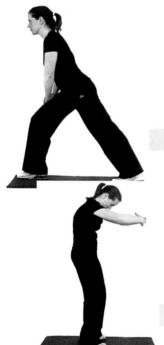

Take a step forward, leaving the heel of the rear foot firmly on the floor as you do. If you cannot feel the stretch, move the rear foot further back until you do.

SOLEUS & ACHILLES TENDON (LOWER CALF AREA)

Stand with one foot in front of the other with only a small gap between them. Lower your hips as you bend your knees slightly.

TRICEPS (BACK OF UPPER ARM)

Stand with feet shoulder-width apart and take your arms behind your head. Hold the elbow of one arm and gently pull it behind your head.

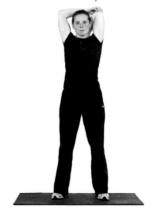

NECK MUSCLES

Place your hand on top of your head, then gently ease the head down toward the shoulder – do not bring the shoulder up to meet it.

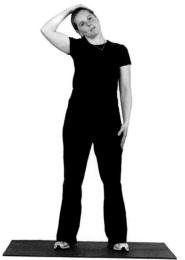

OTHER WAYS TO IMPROVE FLEXIBILITY

Other ways of increasing your flexibility are to go to flexibility classes, such as Pilates, Yoga, Body Balance and so on.

You can work on your flexibility daily, as long as you feel warm you can perform the stretches shown above everyday and within seven days you will notice a difference. The key to enjoying increased mobility and flexibility is to stretch regularly – the old saying 'Use it or lose it!'

EATING RIGHT

In this day and age everybody, even schoolchildren, have a pretty accurate idea about the difference between the kinds of foods that are recommended and encouraged, and those that are unhealthy, or even harmful. We are told to get our "5 a day", cut out fatty foods and, in general, make healthy choices. Whether or not people, armed with this information, will make a healthy choice in the matter is a completely different story. Ironically the unhealthy food, mainly in the form of takeaways and fast food outlets, is chosen because it is regarded as 'cheap' food. In actual fact the cost usually comes not in monetary terms, but in health costs; this stuff can really threaten your state of health, not to mention your waistline. Those people at the infamous 'eat all you can buffet', who appear to be attempting to eat their own bodyweight in food, might think they are getting more value; what, in fact, they are getting is excessively more calories, most of which they will, unfortunately for their health, not be burning off.

The good news is that you don't need to starve yourself to lose weight. You are better off eating to lose weight. The secret is to eat the right foods and cut out the wrong ones. There is so much information available with regard to the difference between intelligent eating and downright stupid eating that nobody can really dispute the fact that they don't know the difference. If you intend to get involved in a training programme it really is wise to evaluate what kind of intake you will need to fuel your body for your workouts – and then stick to it. We are unlikely to put fuel into our car that may harm the engine, so why would anybody want to put fuel into their body that they know is potentially harmful?

It is fairly obvious that our diet has a significant influence on our fitness performance. 'Fad' diets, like those based around cabbage, bananas, grapefruit etc. are a waste of time – how long could a person stay on this kind of diet? What is required is a diet for life, not for a few weeks or months.

A balanced diet, both in quality and quantity before, after, and in some cases, during activity will greatly benefit performance.

In most cases the balance should be:

Carbohydrate 60-70 %

Protein approx. 12%

The remainder will come from fat, which should not exceed 30%.

When it comes to dropping a few pounds, a little research into what you should eat is a good start toward a positive outcome. Expert advice on the subject is not hard to obtain. God only knows how many hours of television time are devoted to it.

The good news is that good foods are, in general, more filling, whereas junk food tends to leave you feeling unfulfilled. So by improving the quality of your intake, you should gradually be satisfied with a smaller volume of food, in which there is a lower percentage of fat, helping you improve your weight. There is no need, however, to eat food you openly dislike or, worse still, have an allergy to; there is a rich variety of good food available in the shape of fruit, vegetables and starchy food (such as bread, cereal, pasta, potatoes, rice), semi-skimmed milk (skimmed milk always makes me feel as if I'm paying a penance), and lean meats.

If you have the time and the ability (or your partner's ability) try to cook and eat at home, as opposed to getting take-aways or eating out on rich foods. This way you are less likely to add excessive salt or artificial additives of the kind the manufacturers include.

Give your heart a break and cut out unnecessary salt from your diet, especially if there is a history of blood pressure or heart disease in your family history. Read food labels and check out the amount of 'sodium'; high levels can be found in salted nuts, crisps and similar snacks, savoury biscuits and 'hidden' in many processed foods such as canned soup, ready-made meals, pickles and sauces and even breakfast cereals. Choose brands with the lowest levels or make your own soups and cereals. Easy guide cookbooks to whip up healthy concoctions that actually taste good have never been more abundant.

When training causes sweat loss to become high it is essential to increase your fluid intake to prevent dehydration. A plastic water bottle to always have by you is one of the smartest investments you can make.

TIMING & TRAINING

Timing your food is important. You need to eat 2-3 hours before you work out, according to how well you digest your food. The meal should incorporate complex carbohydrates. After training you need to elevate your glucose level, if possible within an hour, but if that is not convenient, then as soon as possible. Aim to go for a light meal, rich in carbohydrate.

Always eat breakfast. Cereal and milk are fine if at home. If you have had to dash off and have to find something inexpensive to do the job somewhere as unlikely as McDonalds will be fine if you go for a couple of English muffins with jam, orange juice and an unsweetened cup of tea.

If you have arrived home late and have not eaten, choose something light, such as salad or pasta, so as not to disturb your sleep. Do not go to bed hungry – you might just get up in the night and raid the fridge.

Keep some dried fruit i.e. raisins, apricots or nuts handy for those occasions when you are "absolutely starving".

SPORTS DRINKS AND BARS

Sports bar manufacturers make terrific claims about the energy these bars provide, which they hope will justify the inflated price of so many of them. It is important to read the label and avoid those that are high in fat. A more economical alternative is the cereal bar (or a bowl of cereal and milk if convenient) which should be capable of replacing lost energy just as effectively, especially if teamed with a banana.

DIY Banana Power Shake: You will need one ripe banana, one pint of cold semi-skimmed milk, one low-fat banana yoghurt, one scoop of low fat ice-cream, a handful of ice cubes, a large spoonful of honey (the more you like the taste of honey – the bigger the spoon).

Blend the banana with a small amount of milk, add ice cubes and blend them in. Add the rest of the ingredients and blend on the highest setting. Makes 2-3 good-sized servings.

Any combination of berries can be blended with semi-skimmed milk and low-fat ice cream or yoghurt.

Sports drinks contain carbohydrate and so refuel you more effectively than water. Some people find them unpalatable, particularly the isotonic variety. If you cannot afford or simply dislike the taste of drinks such as Lucozade, Gatorade, Isostar – make your own sports drink and keep it in the fridge.

DIY SPORTS DRINK

Boil a half litre of water, allow to cool. Add a half litre of your favourite pure fruit juice such as orange, pineapple, grapefruit. Add a pinch of salt. Mix well and refrigerate.

Smoothies are nutritious drinks, perfect for refuelling after training. They are usually high in flavour and carbohydrates – but also high in price. You may want to make your own 'power shake' using a blender. I find food processors a pain to wash up afterward and "smoothie makers" no better, but more expensive, than a standard blender.

Salter Essential Blender £16.99

Kenwood Chrome Blender £22.49

Tesco Value Blender £9.77

Four books, from the many available, I would recommend, mostly because of the writers' credentials but also because they are all relatively inexpensive paperbacks:

Nigel Slater's Real Food (Fourth Estate)

The Complete Guide to Sports Nutrition by Anita Bean (A & C Black)

Food For Fitness by Anita Bean (A & C Black)

Sports Nutrition Guidebook by Nancy Clark (Human Kinetics)

FOOD DIARY

A six month study involving 1,685 middle-aged men and women from four U.S. cities showed that keeping a food diary is a great weight- loss aid. The average weight loss of these individuals was about 13lb; the ones who kept food diaries lost about 18lb, compared to 9lb for those who did not keep a diary. The participants were asked to eat less fat and more vegetables, fruit and whole grains; they were also asked to exercise for three hours a week, mostly by walking, and to attend support meetings.

Dr Victor Stevens, of Kaiser Permante's Centre for Health Research in Portland, said "for those who are working on weight loss, just writing down everything you eat is a pretty powerful technique. It helps the participants see where the extra calories are coming from, and then develop more specific plans to deal with those situations."

The study, published in the American Journal of Preventive Medicine, supports earlier research that endorses the value of food diaries in helping dieters lose weight.

(Taken from an article in The Daily Mail, 9th July 2008).

Some years ago I encouraged some people I was training to keep a food diary for what I considered a simple reason — anybody who is trying to lose weight will not want to write down "a Mars Bar", "a jam doughnut", "three pints of lager" if they are even semi-serious about losing some weight, as this would be a record of dismal failure.

The record keeping is for your eyes only (I wouldn't have dreamed of asking to see somebody's food diary any more than their personal diary), so you know if you are staying "on the wagon". If the record is not so good at the start and you have to admit to some less than healthy snacks, you will at least have the chance to put the record straight with minor improvements. The secret is to write down absolutely everything you eat and drink.

What I also did was to suggest keeping an exercise diary to run alongside the food diary. It is not rocket science, or even a very exact science, but it will give you some idea of how to roughly calculate how many calories you have taken in and compare it with those you have expended. (see "Keeping a Record").

INJURY AND ILLNESS

Once you start training, you can get yourself into great shape, but you also run the slight risk of injury, mild or otherwise.

As soon as you feel any pain or marked discomfort – stop training! Rest the painful area immediately, which will reduce circulation, thereby allowing the tissue to begin the repair process. If you don't know what is causing your pain, describe the symptoms to somebody who you think will know, or who is likely to make an educated guess and pass you on to the right channels for treatment.

If your injury turns out to be of a long-term nature it does not necessarily mean you cannot train at all. Do what you can, within the bounds of sound sense and comfort. Leg injuries, according to severity, do not mean you can't still train your upper body, just as something like a sprained wrist or elbow ligament problems will not prevent leg training.

Do not put off getting a chronic problem examined professionally.

Find out how to 'self-help' in the future; if your niggle has been hanging around for a while, do some research into it. The web or the public library is almost certain to have something on the subject.

There are books available to teach you how to do your own massage, which is not as tricky as it may at first appear, and which can, with a little patience, prove very beneficial.

(See "*massage and self-massage*" below).

Make sure you are warm enough when you train outdoors, as cold muscle fibres do not respond well to being extended. On one of those rare blistering hot summer days, cover your head to protect against sunstroke or simply train at a cooler time of day.

When buying any sports shoes, try to do so later in the day when, believe it or not, your feet will be a little larger, by as much as 5%. Tight-fitting shoes can lead to all sorts of foot problems. Blisters are a common problem with people who have recently taken up running for fitness. To prevent them re-occurring, smear the soles of your feet with a coating of Vaseline (petroleum jelly). Treat blisters by dressing them with a 'blister pack', available from pharmacists, and keep them clean to avoid infection if the skin is broken.

CHRONIC PROBLEMS

As stated – if an injury does not show significant improvement with adequate rest and care, or re-occurs when starting training again – seek professional advice.

ILLNESS

There will, inevitably, be times when you will fall prey to the odd cold. The general rule of thumb regarding training is:

If it's from the neck up (sniffles etc.), train lightly.

If it's from the neck down (aching limbs, coughing, wheezing, feeling of lethargy), do not train at all. Wait for the "all clear" before recommencement.

When returning to training after illness or injury, ease your way back into your regime; you cannot catch up on lost time by overworking, so don't try to.

If friends, family or training partners tell you that you look unwell or off-colour, take notice and proceed carefully: you might just be coming down with something.

FIRST AID

Familiarise yourself with the basic procedure to follow if you or a training partner incurs an injury. The very minimum you should know and remember is "RICE".

"R" is for 'rest'. Stop training now!

"I" is for 'ice'. Get some ice, very cold water or freeze-spray applied to the site of the injury as soon as possible, and try to keep it on for 20 minutes every hour. With ice, wrap in a towel first, to prevent ice burn.

"C" is for 'compression'. Apply firm bandage or strapping to prevent painful movement and limit swelling.

"E" is for 'elevation'. Raise the injured limb to allow blood to flow back to the heart.

This is the most basic explanation of "RICE", but this little information is better than nothing, and quite easy to remember and put into effect. Obviously if the injured person is in apparent agony or has suffered a major trauma, do not do anything other than call for an ambulance as quickly as possible, then make them as comfortable as you can while they wait for professional medical assistance.

A one-day first-aid course is relatively inexpensive and many local councils have them running continuously. Attending such a course counts not only for your own welfare in a crisis, but for friends, family and, more usually, total strangers.

TRAIN SENSIBLY

Don't take unnecessary risks like carrying on when in pain, going out running on icy pavements or on foggy evenings.

Never train vigorously in extremes of temperature, especially heat; try to train at the cooler part of the day and ensure you keep your fluid content up.

Try to always get a decent night's sleep, but if you have had a rough, sleepless night don't train too hard the next day.

■ ■ ■ ■ ■ ■ ■ ■ ■ ■ ■ ■ ■ ■ ■ ■ ■ ■ ■ ■

ACHILLES TENDON AND CALF PROBLEMS

The Achilles tendon is a thick, strong band stretching from the calf muscle to the heel. The worst injury in this region is a complete or even partial rupture of the Achilles tendon. Not only is it excruciatingly painful, but walking or even standing becomes impossible. The tendon, if completely ruptured, will need to be repaired by being stitched together (sutured) and then immobilised in a cast or splint for six to eight weeks.

Calf pain is a common problem with runners and can occur for a number of reasons, some avoidable, some which need professional advice to ascertain why they re-occur. The avoidable is usually poor technique or inadequate footwear. Those comfy old trainers may need closer inspection, especially if they have a heel tab that is causing friction, or if the sole is worn and the insole completely worn out. Go to a specialist running shop for a shoe specific to your needs. Decent shoes need not be the most expensive; at the time of writing quality brands including New Balance, Saucony and Brooks all offer shoes priced from **£20-30**.

If you feel the onset of a nagging pain in the calf while out running/ jogging, then slow to a stop and walk to your destination – you cannot 'run it off'. It can aggravate the injury considerably. On reaching home, or the changing room, get some ice on it as quickly as you possibly can. After this carry on the R.I.C.E. procedure and start stretching as soon as the pain subsides, in order to retain flexibility. If walking is difficult try inserting a ready-made heel support (Boots sell these), of sorbothane or supple sponge rubber.

In addition to the calf stretches shown in the chapter on flexibility and stretching, there are other specific calf stretches you can supplement your recovery with:

THE 'DOORSTEP STRETCH'

Supporting your upper body, allow your heels to overhang the edge of a step or stair. Lean forward and allow your heels to drop as low as they can. Hold this for 10-15 seconds.

As before but with your heels turned out to give a pigeon-toed effect.

As before but with the heels closer together in a 'ten to two', Charlie Chaplin stance (for more mature readers).

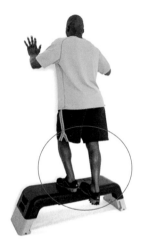 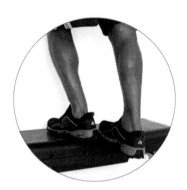

EXERCISE BAND STRETCH

Take an exercise band or a skipping rope and loop it around your foot while seated. While pulling on the band push your toes forward against the resistance. This can also be done with a leather or fabric belt if it is long enough to do the job.

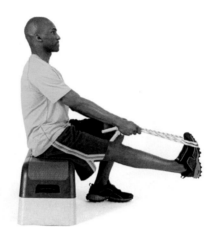

CRAMP

Another calf problem is that of cramp; you can, if you are unfortunate enough, get it in various places, but it is usually as you stretch with effort to reach that forehand ground stroke, make that goal-line clearance or similar. You feel a spasm in the back of your lower leg and realise you are, temporarily at least, out of the action. The usual course of action, often viewed on weekends at park football matches (professionals only seem to get it in cup finals for some reason), is to lay on the ground while somebody holds your heel and forces the sole and toes of your foot downward. Untrained muscles run the highest risk of falling victim to cramp. This technique will most likely relieve the spasm, but, if it continues, a vigorous massage should be tried next. If you have nobody around to manipulate your foot, press your toe against a hard surface, such as a wall or a tree, and lean forward to stretch the calf muscle. If this fails, self-massage comes next. You will need to rub the affected area vigorously, while gritting your teeth, in all likelihood.

The causes of cramp are considered to be a deficit of fluid, salt, calcium or magnesium. Habitual cramp sufferers sometimes prevent its onset by eating a packet of crisps an hour or two before exercise, purely for the salt content. Others swear by eating a banana or a bowl of cereal and milk; if you are a regular cramp sufferer you can experiment to find your cure, but frequent attacks should be discussed with your G.P. in case there is a serious underlying problem involving blood circulation.

SHIN SPLINTS

With this injury pain is felt at the front of the lower leg, along the shinbone. It can often start out as a nagging ache but gradually increase, with activity, into a quite painful and debilitating condition. It is usually caused by landing, during running/jogging, football or other activities involving rebounding, on hard or uneven surfaces. Amateur footballers often sustain this injury at the beginning of the season, when their new boots come in contact with hard grounds, as do novice runners setting out on hard pavements. Technique and footwear should both be carefully scrutinised to prevent re-occurrence once recovery is complete and training is resumed.

Self-help involves using ice as soon as possible. As soon as the pain level allows, start stretching by pulling your toes towards you, preferably against resistance for more effect: sit down and insert your toes under a heavy bench, then extend your legs fully until you feel the effect of the action on the injury site. Alternatively, get a friend, preferably one of slight build, to stand on your toes as you recline, or press against your feet with their hands.

SPRAINS

ANKLE

Sprains are generally caused by the ankle 'going over' on an uneven surface, a stumble when moving quickly, or, in my case, missing the edge of a kerb in bad light. There are, commonly, two types of ankle sprain: damaging either the lateral (outside area), or the medial (inside area).

An inversion injury is likely to injure ligaments on the outside (lateral) side of the ankle. This is the more common injury because there is greater movement in inversion.

An eversion injury is likely to injure ligaments on the inside (medial) side of the ankle. This is less common because there is less movement in eversion.

At first, you may think you have "only twisted your ankle, it might be all right." However, when you arrive home the pain has grown, and so has your ankle – usually to twice the normal size.

Your foot starts to feel hot, and the dull ache becomes sickeningly painful and tender to the touch, and any movement is jarring – yes, it's not just a twist, it's a sprain.

Fill a plastic bowl, or better still, a 'decorators bucket', a rectangular one, that will allow all the foot to fit in fully extended, with cold water and empty the contents of your ice tray into the water. Plunge your foot in – again while gritting your teeth. Failing this, wrap a packet of frozen peas around the affected side and secure with a tea towel or stuffed down a long sock, and rest your injured leg over the arm of the sofa, or similar, for support. From here on follow R.I.C.E. procedure, but it is always worth getting a doctor to look at the injury, who may suspect a fracture and send you for an X-ray to make sure.

Once the swelling and pain subside, usually after about one to two weeks, start to exercise your ankle by rotating in both directions, and with an up and down movement of the foot, to improve mobility and flexibility. Roll a tennis ball around with your bare foot to improve strength and control in the ankle.

WRIST SPRAIN

The wrist is another joint susceptible to sprains, usually incurred by a heavy fall or being wrenched during exercise or working. As before, plunge the affected limb into a bowl or bucket of cold water with a generous helping of ice cubes. As with the ankle it is worth getting a doctor's opinion in case it is not just a sprain, but a fracture.

Once the pain and swelling allow, get the joint moving again and try some wrist strengthening exercises using a small dumbbell or a soup can.

UPWARD ROLL

Hold the weight over the edge of a bench or table, palm facing upward. Slowly bring the hand up towards you, knuckles facing towards you. Try to do *3 sets of 10 repetitions*

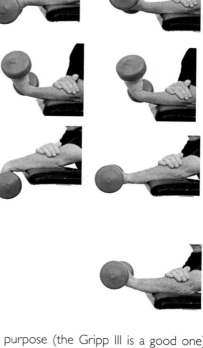

DOWNWARD ROLL

Hold the weight over the edge of the surface with palm facing down. Slowly bring the weight upward as far as you can, with back of the hand facing you. Try to do *3 sets of 10 repetitions*.

Strengthen the muscles of the forearm by investing in a squash ball or one of those squishy sponge balls made for the purpose (the Gripp III is a good one) and carry it in the car to use when sitting in a long wait in traffic, or in your pocket to squeeze while waiting for bus, tube or train, while viewing something mind-numbing on television or reading the newspaper – multi-tasking that works for everybody.

MASSAGE AND SELF MASSAGE

Massage is an ancient healing art and can often achieve outstanding results where other healing has failed. It relaxes tired bodies and eases stiff muscles and joints. A session with a professional masseur/masseuse is wonderful, but if you need regular massage it can become expensive. Home massage is an alternative.

In the list of useful literature I have included "**Sports and Remedial Massage**", by Mel Cash (about **£15**), and "**The Complete Guide to Massage**" by Susan Mumford (at about **£10**); both have a chapter on self-massage, in case you are not in a situation where somebody can give you a massage. The second book is good for total beginners who want to massage or self-massage.

Massage oil can be bought ready-made, but it is equally effective and much cheaper to make your own. Use almond oil or rape seed oil as the carrier oil (the bulk liquid), although baby oil or olive oil will do, and then add the essence of your choice, be it lavender, camomile, peppermint or any from the enormous range available. If you have aching muscles, lemongrass would be a particularly good choice.

The mix: get a plastic bottle that will not leak. You don't want everything in your bag, if you have the oil with you, to reek of essence. Body Shop stores sell empty plastic bottles with a reliable seal at very low cost, as they sensibly recycle all the used bottles customers return; don't feel tempted to use a washed-up shampoo container, as it will almost certainly leak. Fill the bottle up to the shoulders so it's about 80% full, then add 2-3 drips of essence to a small bottle, the kind you could slip in your washbag, or 7-8 drips into a half-litre bottle, and shake vigorously. A half-litre bottle of **rape seed oil** from Sainsbury's, Tesco or similar costs a little over a pound. A small bottle of essence from both of the former, or Body Shop, Holland and

Barrett or any health store costs around **£3**, and lasts for ages. For around **£4** you have a long-term supply of massage oil. All you have to do now is rub it in. A massage book will tell you the exact technique, but if you rub towards the heart until the skin reddens, giving an effect referred to as hyperaemia, that will be a good start; apply the oil to warm hands, then to the area requiring massage. Never apply oil directly to the body.

ICE MASSAGE

You can use this handy little device anywhere on the body, but it is extremely useful on strains in the calf muscle.

Take a Styrofoam cup (one of those that break into thousands of little white balls that get everywhere when crushed), and fill to the brim with cold water.

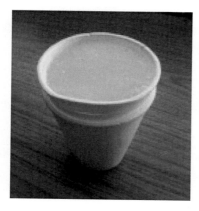

Place the container in your freezer. If the ice has started to split the Styrofoam cup, add a second cup for support. The cups cost **£1** for a large packet in most supermarkets, so you are free to be extravagant with them.

At the first onset of a mildly strained muscle, take the container and cut around the brim with a sharp knife to remove the top half of an inch.

Massage the hard protruding ice around the injured site until the ice softens and becomes unusable. Concentrate solely on the exact site of the injury, don't widen the area that you ice. Time over small areas should be about *5 - 10 minutes.*

Replace cup in freezer. Repeat every time you require it, until it is too small to be practical. For this reason, especially if you are using them regularly, keep two or three in your freezer at the same time.

If the strain is particularly painful, use R.I.C.E. procedure instead.

■ ■ ■ ■ ■ ■ ■ ■ ■ ■ ■ ■ ■ ■ ■ ■ ■

(Sincere thanks to my good friend, osteopath Savash Mustafa, for medical advice in this section).

RECOMMENDED READING;

"Sports Injuries" and "Running Fitness and Injuries", both books by Vivian Grisogono (John Murray)

"Sports Massage" by Dr Jari Ylinen and Mel Cash

"The New Complete Guide to Massage" by Susan Mumford (Hamlyn)

Indispensable Reading: "The St John Ambulance Association and British Red Cross 'First Aid Manual' (Dorling Kindersley)

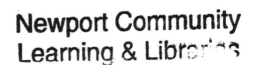